\疾患別/
歯学英単語1000

近藤真治　著

クインテッセンス出版株式会社　2017
QUINTESSENCE PUBLISHING
Berlin, Barcelona, Chicago, Istanbul, London, Milan, Moscow, New Delhi, Paris, Prague, São Paulo, Seoul, Singapore, Tokyo, Warsaw

クインテッセンス出版の書籍・雑誌は、歯学書専用通販サイト『**歯学書.COM**』にてご購入いただけます。

PCからのアクセスは…

歯学書　検索

携帯電話からのアクセスは…
QRコードからモバイルサイトへ

はじめに

　現代は経済，政治，文化など，社会のあらゆる側面でグローバル化が急速に進んでいる時代であるといえます．国際的な情報伝達手段としての英語の重要性はかつてないほど高まっており，英語の学び方や活用の仕方についての本が数多く出版されています．このことは医療の分野においても同様で，いわゆる医療英語に関する参考書や語学教材はかなりの数にのぼります．その一方で，歯学の分野に特化した英語教材は非常に少ないのが現状です．

　歯学英語を学ぶ手段として，英文で書かれた教科書を読んでいる人もいると思われます．教科書は，その分野で使用される用語や表現の宝庫です．ただし，通常数百ページにもわたる英文を，辞書を引き引き読み進める労力を考えると，多くの人が尻込みしてしまうのも事実でしょう．

　専門誌や学会，インターネット等を通じて海外のさまざまな症例を英語で学びたいと考えている歯学関係者の方は多いと思います．本書はそのようなニーズを出発点として企画されました．執筆にあたっては，まず「症例報告の理解に必要不可欠な用語や表現を，英語で効率的に学ぶにはどうすれば良いか」という問いを立ててみました．英文の教科書では敷居が高すぎるのであれば，その内容を精選・凝縮し，さらに和訳を加えれば学習者の負担は大幅に軽減されるはずです．その考えを推し進めた結果，歯学分野における 250 の基本疾患とその定義を英語と日本語で記述するという形に到達しました．本書の学習者は「埋伏歯」，「交叉咬合」，「根尖性歯周炎」等の基本用語・概念を英語で理解し，かつ説明する能力を辞書の助けを借りずに訓練することができます．また，その過程で「萌出する（erupt）」，「唇側の（labial）」，「偏位（deviation）」，「歯周組織（periodontal tissue）」，「炎症（inflammation）」といった関連語やそれらが使用される文脈も

同時に学ぶことができます．掲載されている単語の種類，表現の豊富さの両面において，歯学英語の基礎は本書1冊で十分であると考えています．学習者の皆さんには，何度も本書をめくって，さまざまなセクションのあいだを渡り歩いてみることをお勧めします．本書をめくる回数に比例して，歯学英語の力がついていくのが実感できることでしょう．

　本書を執筆する際,『歯科医師国家試験出題基準』（厚生労働省),『標準口腔外科学』（医学書院),『常用歯科辞典』（医歯薬出版株式会社),『The Merck Manual』（Merck Sharp & Dohme Corp.),『医学書院 医学大辞典』（医学書院),『ステッドマン医学大辞典』（メジカルビュー社),『Stedman's Medical Dictionary』（Lippincott Williams&Wilkins),『医学英和辞典』（研究社）等を参照しました．本書を歯科医師や歯学研究者をはじめ，歯学部学生や大学院生，さらには歯学関連の業務に従事している社会人等の幅広い方がたに利用していただきたいと考えています．

2017年10月

愛知医科大学看護学部教授
近藤真治

Contents

本書の構成 6
1. 歯の異常 12
2. 不正咬合 22
3. 歯の硬組織疾患 27
4. 歯髄・歯周組織疾患 32
5. 顎・口腔領域の先天異常と変形 40
6. 軟組織の炎症 49
7. 囊胞性疾患 54
8. 腫瘍および腫瘍類似疾患 65
9. 口腔粘膜疾患 78
10. 骨の疾患 97
11. 顎関節疾患 100
12. 唾液腺疾患 106
13. 神経疾患 111
14. 歯・口腔・顎顔面に異常を来す疾患・症候群 117
索引 134

本書の構成

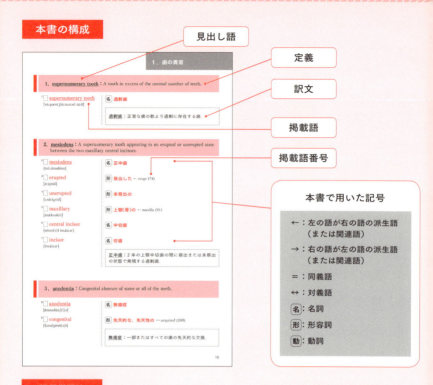

推奨学習法

Step1：見出し語と定義を読む
　見出し語と定義を学習する際は，単語1語ずつの意味と英文全体の構造が完全に理解できるようになるまで，英語と日本語を何度も見比べてください．赤字で掲載されている単語にはとくに注意を払いましょう．一通り学習したら，日本語部分を隠した状態で英語部分を和訳してみてください．この時，声を出して和訳するのがポイントです．この学習により，症例報告や医学書を英語で読む力がおおいに向上するはずです．

Step2：掲載語（赤字の単語）を覚える
　Step 1で和訳の学習が終了したので，次は掲載語を日本語から英語に変換する訓練を行います．それぞれの単語について，発音記号を見ながら音読し，何度も紙に書いて体に覚えこませます．日本語から英語にスムーズに変換できるようになったら，チェックボックスにチェックを入れましょう．

Step3：日本語の定義を英語に変換する
　最後のステップは日本語の定義の英訳です．英文を隠した状態で日本語を英語に直せるようになるのが目標です．このステップはかなりハードルが高いので，比較的簡単な文，あるいは自分が興味のある部分を選んで少しずつ行うようにしましょう．英語で症例報告を書いたり，国際学会で発表したりする人にはお勧めの学習法です．

〈見出し語一覧〉

No	英語	日本語
1. 歯の異常		
1	supernumerary tooth	過剰歯
2	mesiodens	正中歯
3	anodontia	無歯症
4	fused teeth	癒合歯
5	concrescent teeth	癒着歯
6	geminated tooth	双生歯
7	Carabelli's tubercle	カラベリー結節
8	protostylid	プロトスタイリッド
9	dens in dente	歯内歯
10	microdont	矮小歯
11	macrodont	巨大歯
12	conical tooth	円錐歯
13	taurodont	タウロドント
14	enamel drop	エナメル滴
15	fluorosis	フッ素症
16	enamel hypoplasia	エナメル質減形成（症）
17	Turner tooth	ターナー歯
18	Hutchinson teeth	ハッチンソン歯
19	Fournier teeth	フルニエ歯
20	transversion	転位
21	impacted tooth	埋伏歯
22	submerged tooth	低位歯
23	congenital tooth	先天歯
24	delayed eruption	萌出遅延
2. 不正咬合		
25	malocclusion	不正咬合
26	crossbite	交叉咬合
27	open bite	開咬症
28	edge-to-edge occlusion	切端咬合
29	overclosure	低位咬合
30	overbite	過蓋咬合
31	crowding	叢生
32	maxillary protrusion	上顎前突症
33	mandibular protrusion	下顎前突症
34	bimaxillary protrusion	上下顎前突
35	mandibular retrusion	下顎後退症

No	英語	日本語
3. 歯の硬組織疾患		
36	dental caries	う蝕
37	attrition	咬耗症
38	abrasion	摩耗症
39	erosion	酸蝕症
40	abfraction	アブフラクション
41	wedge-shaped defect	くさび状欠損
42	fracture	破折
43	luxation	脱臼
4. 歯髄・歯周組織疾患		
44	dentin hypersensitivity	象牙質知覚過敏症
45	denticle	象牙質粒
46	pulp hyperemia	歯髄充血
47	pulpitis	歯髄炎
48	pulp necrosis	歯髄壊死
49	root resorption	歯根吸収
50	apical periodontitis	根尖性歯周炎
51	gingivitis	歯肉炎
52	desquamative gingivitis	剝離性歯肉炎
53	necrotizing ulcerative gingivitis	壊死性潰瘍性歯肉炎
54	gingival abscess	歯肉膿瘍
55	dental fistula	歯瘻
56	chronic periodontitis	慢性歯周炎
57	occlusal trauma	咬合性外傷
58	gingival recession	歯肉退縮
5. 顎・口腔領域の先天異常と変形		
59	cleft lip	口唇裂
60	alveolar cleft	歯槽裂，顎裂
61	cleft palate	口蓋裂
62	facial cleft	顔面裂
63	submucous cleft palate	粘膜下口蓋裂
64	congenital velopharyngeal insufficiency	先天性鼻咽腔閉鎖不全症
65	macrocheilia	巨唇症
66	double lip	二重唇
67	microstomia	小口症

No	英語	日本語
68	masseter muscle hypertrophy	咬筋肥大症
69	macroglossia	巨舌症
70	microglossia	小舌症
71	cleft tongue	舌裂
72	lingual thyroid	舌甲状腺
73	epithelial pearls	上皮真珠
74	gingival fibromatosis	歯肉線維腫症
75	gingival hyperplasia	歯肉増殖
76	high-arched palate	高口蓋
77	ankyloglossia	舌小帯短縮症
6．軟組織の炎症		
78	pericoronitis	歯冠周囲炎，智歯周囲炎
79	cellulitis	蜂窩織炎，蜂巣炎
80	Ludwig's angina	ルートヴィヒアンギナ
81	odontogenic peritonsillitis	歯性扁桃周囲炎
82	odontogenic maxillary sinusitis	歯性上顎洞炎
83	actinomycosis	放線菌症
84	lupus vulgaris	尋常性狼瘡
85	tuberculous cervical lymphadenitis	結核性頸部リンパ節炎
7．囊胞性疾患		
86	primordial cyst	原始性囊胞
87	odontogenic keratocyst	歯原性角化囊胞
88	dentigerous cyst	含歯性囊胞
89	eruption cyst	萌出囊胞
90	lateral periodontal cyst	側方性歯周囊胞
91	gingival cyst	歯肉囊胞
92	glandular odontogenic cyst	腺性歯原性囊胞
93	nasopalatine duct cyst	鼻口蓋管囊胞
94	nasoalveolar cyst	鼻歯槽囊胞
95	radicular cyst	歯根囊胞
96	residual cyst	残留囊胞

No	英語	日本語
97	paradental cyst	歯周囊胞
98	simple bone cyst	単純性骨囊胞
99	aneurysmal bone cyst	脈瘤性骨囊胞
100	static bone cavity	静止性骨空洞
101	mucous cyst	粘液囊胞
102	ranula	ガマ腫
103	Blandin-Nuhn cyst	ブランダン・ヌーン囊胞
104	dermoid cyst	類皮囊胞
105	epidermoid cyst	類表皮囊胞
106	thyroglossal duct cyst	甲状舌管囊胞
107	branchial cyst	鰓囊胞
108	postoperative maxillary cyst	術後性上顎囊胞
8．腫瘍および腫瘍類似疾患		
109	ameloblastoma	エナメル上皮腫
110	keratocystic odontogenic tumor	角化囊胞性歯原性腫瘍
111	adenomatoid odontogenic tumor	腺腫様歯原性腫瘍
112	calcifying epithelial odontogenic tumor	石灰化上皮性歯原性腫瘍
113	ameloblastic fibroma	エナメル上皮線維腫
114	odontoma	歯牙腫
115	calcifying cystic odontogenic tumor	石灰化囊胞性歯原性腫瘍
116	odontogenic fibroma	歯原性線維腫
117	odontogenic myxoma	歯原性粘液腫
118	cementoblastoma	セメント芽細胞腫
119	primary intraosseous squamous cell carcinoma	原発性骨内扁平上皮癌
120	ameloblastic fibrosarcoma	エナメル上皮線維肉腫
121	pleomorphic adenoma	多形腺腫
122	Warthin tumor	ウォーシン腫瘍
123	oncocytoma	オンコサイトーマ
124	benign lymphoepithelial lesion	良性リンパ上皮性病変

No	英語	日本語
125	chronic sclerosing submandibular sialadenitis	慢性硬化性顎下腺炎
126	oral cancer	口腔癌
127	adenoid cystic carcinoma	腺様嚢胞癌
128	mucoepidermoid carcinoma	粘表皮癌
129	acinic cell carcinoma	腺房細胞癌
130	epulis	エプーリス
131	denture fibroma	義歯性線維腫
132	palatal torus	口蓋隆起
133	mandibular torus	下顎隆起
134	osseous dysplasia	骨性異形成症
135	McCune-Albright syndrome	マッキューン・オールブライト症候群
136	cherubism	ケルビズム
137	Langerhans cell histiocytosis	ランゲルハンス細胞組織球症

9. 口腔粘膜疾患

No	英語	日本語
138	herpetic gingivostomatitis	ヘルペス性歯肉口内炎，疱疹性歯肉口内炎
139	herpes labialis	口唇ヘルペス
140	herpes zoster	帯状疱疹
141	herpangina	ヘルパンギーナ
142	hand-foot-and-mouth disease	手足口病
143	Koplik spots	コプリック斑
144	pemphigus	天疱瘡
145	pemphigoid	類天疱瘡
146	epidermolysis bullosa	表皮水疱症
147	erythema multiforme	多形紅斑
148	Stevens-Johnson syndrome	スティーヴンス・ジョンソン症候群
149	toxic epidermal necrolysis (TEN)	中毒性表皮壊死症
150	systemic lupus erythematosus (SLE)	全身性エリテマトーデス
151	discoid lupus erythematosus (DLE)	円板状エリテマトーデス
152	angioedema	血管性浮腫
153	recurrent aphthous stomatitis	再発性アフタ性口内炎
154	Behçet disease	ベーチェット病
155	gangrenous stomatitis	壊疽性口内炎
156	stomatitis medicamentosa	薬物性口内炎
157	oral lichen planus	口腔扁平苔癬
158	oral candidiasis	口腔カンジダ症
159	leukoplakia	白板症
160	erythroplakia	紅板症
161	hairy leukoplakia	毛状白板症
162	nicotine stomatitis	ニコチン性口内炎
163	melanism	メラニン沈着
164	nevus pigmentosus	色素性母斑
165	Addison's disease	アジソン病
166	angular stomatitis	口角びらん
167	Plummer-Vinson syndrome	プランマー・ヴィンソン症候群
168	Hunter's glossitis	ハンター舌炎
169	fissured tongue	溝状舌
170	black hairy tongue	黒毛舌
171	geographic tongue	地図状舌
172	median rhomboid glossitis	正中菱形舌炎
173	Fordyce spots	フォーダイス斑
174	lingual tonsil hypertrophy	舌扁桃肥大
175	cheilitis	口唇炎
176	granulomatous cheilitis	肉芽腫性口唇炎
177	Melkersson-Rosenthal syndrome	メルカーソン・ローゼンタール症候群
178	contact cheilitis	接触性口唇炎
179	Riga-Fede disease	リガ・フェーデ病
180	Bednar's aphthae	ベドナー・アフタ

No	英語	日本語
10. 骨の疾患		
181	alveolar osteitis	歯槽骨炎
182	periostitis	骨膜炎
183	osteomyelitis	骨髄炎
184	bisphosphonate-related osteonecrosis of the jaw (BRONJ)	ビスフォスフォネート関連顎骨壊死
11. 顎関節疾患		
185	mandibular condylar hyperplasia	下顎頭過形成
186	temporomandibular joint disorder	顎関節症
187	osteoarthritis	変形性関節症
188	traumatic arthritis	外傷性関節炎
189	suppurative arthritis	化膿性関節炎
190	Costen syndrome	コステン症候群
191	rheumatoid arthritis	関節リウマチ
192	gout	痛風
193	articular chondrocalcinosis	関節軟骨石灰化症
194	osteochondroma	骨軟骨腫
195	synovial chondromatosis	滑膜軟骨腫症
196	ankylosis	関節強直
12. 唾液腺疾患		
197	accessory salivary gland	副唾液腺
198	aberrant salivary gland	迷入唾液腺
199	salivary fistula	唾液瘻
200	xerostomia	口腔乾燥症
201	sialorrhea	流涎症
202	sialadenitis	唾液腺炎
203	sialoangiitis	唾液管炎
204	epidemic parotitis	流行性耳下腺炎
205	Mikulicz disease	ミクリッツ病
206	Sjögren syndrome	シェーグレン症候群
207	Frey syndrome	フライ症候群

No	英語	日本語
208	sialolithiasis	唾石症
209	necrotizing sialometaplasia	壊死性唾液腺化生
13. 神経疾患		
210	trigeminal neuralgia	三叉神経痛
211	glossopharyngeal neuralgia	舌咽神経痛
212	complex regional pain syndrome (CRPS)	複合性局所疼痛症候群
213	glossodynia	舌痛症
214	facial paralysis	顔面神経麻痺
215	Ramsay Hunt syndrome	ラムゼイ・ハント症候群
216	Bell's palsy	ベル麻痺
217	facial spasm	顔面痙攣
218	oral dyskinesia	口腔ジスキネジア
219	dysgeusia	味覚異常
14. 歯・口腔・頭顔面に異常を来す疾患・症候群		
220	cleidocranial dysplasia	鎖骨頭蓋異形成症
221	osteopetrosis	大理石骨病
222	osteogenesis imperfecta	骨形成不全症
223	Treacher Collins syndrome	トリーチャー・コリンズ症候群
224	Crouzon syndrome	クルーゾン症候群
225	Apert syndrome	アペール症候群
226	achondroplasia	軟骨無形成症
227	first and second branchial arch syndrome	第一第二鰓弓症候群
228	Goldenhar syndrome	ゴールデンハー症候群
229	oral-facial-digital syndrome	口腔顔面指趾症候群
230	Marfan syndrome	マルファン症候群
231	basal cell nevus syndrome	基底細胞母斑症候群

No	英語	日本語
232	Peutz-Jeghers syndrome	ポイツ・ジェガース症候群
233	Gardner syndrome	ガードナー症候群
234	von Recklinghausen's disease	フォン・レックリングハウゼン病
235	Sturge-Weber syndrome	スタージ・ウェーバー症候群
236	Russell-Silver syndrome	ラッセル・シルヴァー症候群
237	Turner syndrome	ターナー症候群
238	Beckwith-Wiedemann syndrome	ベックウィズ・ヴィーデマン症候群
239	Pierre Robin syndrome	ピエール・ロバン症候群
240	amelogenesis imperfecta	エナメル質形成不全症

No	英語	日本語
241	dentinogenesis imperfecta	象牙質形成不全症
242	dentin dysplasia	象牙質異形成症
243	congenital ectodermal dysplasia	先天性外胚葉形成不全，先天性外胚葉異形成症
244	incontinentia pigmenti	色素失調症
245	hypophosphatasia	低フォスファターゼ症
246	Papillon-Lefèvre syndrome	パピヨン・ルフェーヴル症候群
247	Down syndrome	ダウン症候群
248	Klinefelter syndrome	クラインフェルター症候群
249	trisomy 18 syndrome	18トリソミー症候群
250	cri du chat syndrome	猫鳴き症候群

1 | 歯の異常

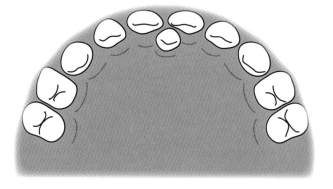

1. 歯の異常

1. <u>supernumerary tooth</u>：A tooth in excess of the normal number of teeth.

1. ☐ <u>supernumerary tooth</u>
[sùːpərn(j)úːmərəri túːθ]

名 過剰歯

> <u>過剰歯</u>：正常な歯の数より過剰に存在する歯．

2. <u>mesiodens</u>：A supernumerary tooth appearing in an erupted or unerupted state between the two maxillary central incisors.

2. ☐ <u>mesiodens</u>
[míːzioudènz]

名 正中歯

3. ☐ erupted
[irʌ́ptid]

形 萌出した ← erupt (74)

4. ☐ unerupted
[ʌnirʌ́ptid]

形 未萌出の

5. ☐ maxillary
[mǽksəlèri]

形 上顎(骨)の ← maxilla (91)

6. ☐ central incisor
[séntr(ə)l insáizər]

名 中切歯

7. ☐ incisor
[insáizər]

名 切歯

> <u>正中歯</u>：2本の上顎中切歯の間に萌出または未萌出の状態で発現する過剰歯．

3. <u>anodontia</u>：Congenital absence of some or all of the teeth.

8. ☐ <u>anodontia</u>
[ænoudánʃ(i)ə]

名 無歯症

9. ☐ congenital
[kəndʒénit(ə)l]

形 先天的な，先天性の ↔ acquired (240)

> <u>無歯症</u>：一部またはすべての歯の先天的な欠損．

1. 歯の異常

4. **fused teeth**: Teeth joined by dentin through union of two adjacent tooth germs.

10 ☐ fused teeth [fjú:zd tí:θ] 名 癒合歯

11 ☐ dentin [déntən] 名 象牙質

12 ☐ tooth germ [tú:θ dʒə́:rm] 名 歯胚

癒合歯:2つの隣り合う歯胚の一体化により象牙質が結合した歯.

5. **concrescent teeth**: Teeth joined by cementum after the dentin formation is completed.

13 ☐ concrescent teeth [kɑnkrésənt tí:θ] 名 癒着歯

14 ☐ cementum [səméntəm] 名 セメント質

癒着歯:象牙質形成が完了した後にセメント質が結合した歯.

6. **geminated tooth**: A tooth with two partially or completely separated crowns on a single root.

15 ☐ geminated tooth [dʒémənèitid tú:θ] 名 双生歯

16 ☐ crown [kráun] 名 歯冠

17 ☐ root [rú:t] 名 歯根

双生歯:1つの歯根の上に部分的または完全に分離した2つの歯冠をもつ歯.

1. 歯の異常

7. <u>Carabelli's tubercle</u>：A tubercle found on the lingual surface of the mesiolingual cusp of maxillary molars.

18 ☐ <u>Carabelli's tubercle</u>
[kà:ra:béliz t(j)ú:bərk(ə)l]

|名| カラベリー結節

19 ☐ tubercle
[t(j)ú:bərk(ə)l]

|名| 結節

20 ☐ lingual
[líŋwəl]

|形| 舌側の

21 ☐ mesiolingual
[mì:zioulíŋwəl]

|形| 近心舌側の

22 ☐ cusp
[kʌ́sp]

|名| 咬頭

23 ☐ molar
[móulər]

|名| 大臼歯

> カラベリー結節：上顎大臼歯の近心舌側咬頭の舌側面に見られる結節．

8. <u>protostylid</u>：A tubercle found on the buccal surface of the mesiobuccal cusp of mandibular molars.

24 ☐ <u>protostylid</u>
[pròutoustáiləd]

|名| プロトスタイリッド

25 ☐ buccal
[bʌ́k(ə)l]

|形| 頬側の

26 ☐ mesiobuccal
[mì:zioubʌ́k(ə)l]

|形| 近心頬側の

27 ☐ mandibular
[mændíbjələr]

|形| 下顎(骨)の ← mandible (93)

> プロトスタイリッド：下顎大臼歯の近心頬側咬頭の頬側面に見られる結節．

1. 歯の異常

9. dens in dente: Malformation of the teeth, found chiefly in the maxillary lateral incisors, in which coronal enamel and dentin are invaginated into the pulp cavity.

28 **dens in dente** [dénz in dénti] 名 歯内歯

29 **malformation** [mæ̀lfɔːrméiʃ(ə)n] 名 奇形

30 **lateral** [lǽtər(ə)l] 形 外側の ↔ medial (210)

31 **lateral incisor** [lǽtər(ə)l insáizər] 名 側切歯

32 **coronal** [kɔ́rən(ə)l] 形 歯冠(部)の

33 **enamel** [inǽm(ə)l] 名 エナメル質

34 **invaginate** [invǽdʒənèit] 動 陥入する

35 **pulp cavity** [pʌ́lp kǽvəti] 名 歯髄腔

歯内歯：主に上顎側切歯に見られる歯の奇形．歯冠部のエナメル質と象牙質が歯髄腔内に陥入している．

10. microdont: An abnormally small tooth.

36 **microdont** [máikrədùnt] 名 矮小歯 → microdontia (985)

矮小歯：異常に小さな歯．

11. macrodont: An abnormally large tooth.

37 **macrodont** [mǽkrədùnt] 名 巨大歯 → macrodontia (986)

巨大歯：異常に大きな歯．

1. 歯の異常

12. conical tooth (=peg tooth): A tooth with a crown diameter that decreases from cervical margin to incisal edge.

38 conical tooth [kánik(ə)l túːθ]	名 円錐歯
39 peg tooth [pég túːθ]	名 栓状歯
40 cervical [sə́ːrvik(ə)l]	形 歯頸(部)の，頸部の
41 cervical margin [sə́ːrvik(ə)l máːrdʒən]	名 歯頸縁
42 incisal edge [insáiz(ə)l édʒ]	名 切縁

> **円錐歯(＝栓状歯)**：歯頸縁から切縁にかけて歯冠の直径が減少した歯．

---

13. taurodont: A tooth with an enlarged pulp cavity and reduced roots.

43 taurodont [tɔ́ːrədànt]	名 タウロドント

> **タウロドント**：歯髄腔が拡大し歯根が短縮した歯．

---

14. enamel drop (=enamel pearl): A spherical nodule of enamel below the cementoenamel junction, usually at the bifurcation of molars.

44 enamel drop [inǽm(ə)l dráp]	名 エナメル滴
45 enamel pearl [inǽm(ə)l pə́ːrl]	名 エナメル真珠
46 nodule [nádʒùːl]	名 小結節
47 cementoenamel junction [simèntouinǽm(ə)l dʒʌ́ŋkʃ(ə)n]	名 セメントエナメル境

1. 歯の異常

⁴⁸ **bifurcation**
[bàifərkéiʃ(ə)n]

名 分岐部

> **エナメル滴（＝エナメル真珠）**：エナメルセメント境より下位，通常は大臼歯の歯根分岐部に見られるエナメル質の球状の小結節．

15. fluorosis : A condition caused by an excessive intake of fluorine or its compounds, characterized by hypoplasia of the enamel and mottled teeth.

⁴⁹ **fluorosis**
[flùəróusəs]

名 フッ素症

⁵⁰ **fluorine**
[flúərì:n]

名 フッ素

⁵¹ **compound**
[kámpàund]

名 化合物

⁵² **hypoplasia**
[hàipoupléiʒ(i)ə]

名 形成不全，減形成

⁵³ **mottled tooth**
[mátld tú:θ]

名 斑状歯

> **フッ素症**：フッ素またはその化合物の過剰摂取に起因する症状．エナメル質の形成不全と斑状歯を特徴とする．

16. enamel hypoplasia : A developmental disorder of teeth characterized by deficient enamel matrix formation, caused by fluorosis, malnutrition, childhood fevers, or congenital syphilis.

⁵⁴ **enamel hypoplasia**
[inæm(ə)l hàipoupléiʒ(i)ə]

名 エナメル質減形成（症）

⁵⁵ **developmental disorder**
[divèləpmént(ə)l disɔ́:rdər]

名 発育障害

⁵⁶ **matrix**
[méitriks]

名 基質

⁵⁷ **malnutrition**
[mæ̀ln(j)u:tríʃ(ə)n]

名 栄養不良

⁵⁸ **fever**
[fí:vər]

名 発熱

1. 歯の異常

59 ☐ **syphilis**
[sífələs]

名 梅毒

エナメル質減形成(症)：エナメル質基質の形成不全を特徴とする歯の発育障害．フッ素症，栄養不良，小児期の発熱，先天梅毒等に起因する．

---

17. Turner tooth：Enamel hypoplasia involving a permanent tooth, caused by inflammation in the deciduous tooth that preceded it or to trauma during odontogenesis.

60 ☐ **Turner tooth**
[tə́ːrnər túːθ]

名 ターナー歯

61 ☐ **permanent tooth**
[pə́ːrmənənt túːθ]

名 永久歯 ↔ deciduous tooth (63)

62 ☐ **inflammation**
[ìnfləméiʃ(ə)n]

名 炎症

63 ☐ **deciduous tooth**
[disídʒuəs túːθ]

名 乳歯 ↔ permanent tooth (61)

64 ☐ **trauma**
[trɔ́ːmə]

名 外傷

65 ☐ **odontogenesis**
[oudàntoudʒénəsəs]

名 歯牙形成

ターナー歯：永久歯に生じるエナメル質減形成．以前に生えていた乳歯の炎症や歯牙形成期の外傷に起因する．

---

18. Hutchinson teeth：Malformation of maxillary central incisors seen in congenital syphilis in which the incisal edge is notched and narrower than the cervical area.

66 ☐ **Hutchinson teeth**
[hʌ́tʃənsən tíːθ]

名 ハッチンソン歯

67 ☐ **notched**
[nɑ́tʃt]

形 切痕のある

ハッチンソン歯：先天梅毒に見られる上顎中切歯の奇形．切縁に切痕があり，歯頸部より幅が狭い．

1. 歯の異常

19. <u>Fournier teeth</u> (=<u>Moon teeth</u>)：Mulberry-like malformation of first molars seen in congenital syphilis characterized by a dome-shaped crown and dwarfed cusps.

68 ☐ <u>Fournier teeth</u>
[fùːrnjéi tíːθ]

【名】フルニエ歯

69 ☐ <u>Moon teeth</u>
[múːn tíːθ]

【名】ムーン歯

70 ☐ first molar
[fə́ːrst móulər]

【名】第一大臼歯

<u>フルニエ歯（＝ムーン歯）</u>：先天梅毒に見られる第一大臼歯の桑実様の奇形で，ドーム状の歯冠と萎縮した咬頭を特徴とする．

---

20. <u>transversion</u>：Misplacement of teeth from normal sequence in the dental arch.

71 ☐ transversion
[trænsvə́ːrʒ(ə)n]

【名】転位

72 ☐ dental arch
[dént(ə)l áːrtʃ]

【名】歯列弓

<u>転位</u>：歯列弓上の正常な並びからの歯の偏位．

---

21. <u>impacted tooth</u>：A tooth that is prevented from erupting by adjacent teeth, bone, or tissue.

73 ☐ <u>impacted tooth</u>
[impǽktid túːθ]

【名】埋伏歯

74 ☐ erupt
[irʌ́pt]

【動】萌出する

75 ☐ tissue
[tíʃu]

【名】組織

<u>埋伏歯</u>：隣接する歯，骨，組織等によって萌出が妨げられている歯．

1. 歯の異常

22. <u>submerged tooth</u>: A deciduous tooth that is below the occlusal plane.

76 □ <u>submerged tooth</u>
[səbmə́:rdʒd túːθ]

77 □ occlusal
[əklúːs(ə)l]

78 □ occlusal plane
[əklúːs(ə)l pléin]

名 低位歯

形 咬合の ← occlusion (95)

名 咬合平面

> <u>低位歯</u>：咬合平面より低位にある乳歯．

23. <u>congenital tooth</u>: A tooth that has erupted at birth or erupts during the neonatal period.

79 □ <u>congenital tooth</u>
[kəndʒénit(ə)l túːθ]

80 □ neonatal
[nìːənéit(ə)l]

名 先天歯

形 新生児の ← neonate (260)

> <u>先天歯</u>：出産時に既に萌出している，または新生児期に萌出する歯．

24. <u>delayed eruption</u>: Dental eruption that is chronologically later than normal.

81 □ <u>delayed eruption</u>
[diléid irʌ́pʃ(ə)n]

82 □ eruption
[irʌ́pʃ(ə)n]

名 萌出遅延 ↔ early eruption (987)

名 萌出 ← erupt (74)

> <u>萌出遅延</u>：歯の萌出が正常より時期的に遅いこと．

2 | 不正咬合

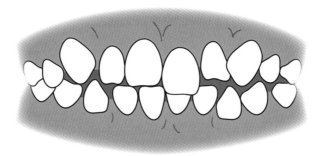

2．不正咬合

25. <u>malocclusion</u>： Abnormal contact between the teeth of the upper jaw and those of the lower jaw.

83 ☐ <u>malocclusion</u>
[mæləklúːʒ(ə)n]

名 不正咬合

84 ☐ jaw
[dʒɔ́ː]

名 顎（骨）

> <u>不正咬合</u>：上顎の歯と下顎の歯の噛み合わせの異常．

26. <u>crossbite</u>： Malocclusion due to labial, buccal, or lingual deviation of tooth position, or to abnormal jaw position.

85 ☐ <u>crossbite</u>
[krɔ́sbàit]

名 交叉咬合

86 ☐ labial
[léibiəl]

形 唇側の

87 ☐ deviation
[dìːviéiʃ(ə)n]

名 偏位

> <u>交叉咬合</u>：歯の唇側・頬側・舌側への偏位または顎の位置の異常に起因する不正咬合．

27. <u>open bite</u>： A condition in which some teeth, especially anterior teeth, in the maxilla do not contact the opposing teeth in the mandible in centric occlusion.

88 ☐ <u>open bite</u>
[óupən báit]

名 開咬症

89 ☐ anterior
[æntíəriər]

形 前方の ↔ posterior (110)

90 ☐ anterior teeth
[æntíəriər tíːθ]

名 前歯

91 ☐ maxilla
[mæksílə]

名 上顎（骨）

92 ☐ opposing teeth
[əpóuziŋ tíːθ]

名 対合歯

93 ☐ mandible
[mǽndəbl]

名 下顎（骨）

2. 不正咬合

94 **centric occlusion**
[séntrik əklúːʒ(ə)n]

名 中心咬合位

95 **occlusion**
[əklúːʒ(ə)n]

名 咬合

> <u>開咬症</u>：中心咬合位において上顎の歯，とくに前歯が下顎の対合歯に接触しない状態．

28. <u>edge-to-edge occlusion</u>：A condition in which the anterior teeth of both jaws meet along their incisal edges in centric occlusion.

96 <u>edge-to-edge occlusion</u>
[édʒ tu: édʒ əklúːʒ(ə)n]

名 切端咬合

> <u>切端咬合</u>：中心咬合位において上下顎の前歯がその切縁で接している状態．

29. <u>overclosure</u>：A decrease in occlusal vertical dimension caused by drifting of teeth, change in tooth shapes through grinding, or loss of teeth.

97 <u>overclosure</u>
[òuvərklóuʒər]

名 低位咬合

98 **occlusal vertical dimension**
[əklúːsəl vəːrtik(ə)l dəménʃ(ə)n]

名 咬合高径

99 **drifting**
[dríftiŋ]

名 移動（歯がより安定な位置へ向かって移動すること）

> <u>低位咬合</u>：歯の移動，摩耗による歯形の変化，歯の欠損等に起因する咬合高径の減少．

30. <u>overbite</u>：Vertical overlapping of the mandibular anterior teeth by the maxillary anterior teeth.

100 <u>overbite</u>
[óuvərbàit]

名 過蓋咬合

> <u>過蓋咬合</u>：上顎前歯が下顎前歯に垂直的にかぶさっている状態．

2．不正咬合

31. crowding：A condition in which teeth are crowded and have abnormal positions such as overlapping and torsiversion.

101 □ **crowding**
[kráudiŋ]

名 叢生

102 □ **torsiversion**
[tɔ̀ːrsəvə́ːrʒ(ə)n]

名 捻転

> <u>叢生</u>：歯が異常な位置に混み合って生えている状態で，重なり合いや捻転が見られる．

32. maxillary protrusion：An abnormal anterior positioning of the maxilla relative to the facial skeleton.

103 □ **maxillary protrusion**
[mǽksəlèri proutrúːʒ(ə)n]

名 上顎前突症

104 □ **skeleton**
[skélətən]

名 骨格

> <u>上顎前突症</u>：顔面骨格に対して上顎骨が異常に前突していること．

33. mandibular protrusion：An abnormal anterior positioning of the mandible relative to the facial skeleton.

105 □ **mandibular protrusion**
[mændíbjələr proutrúːʒ(ə)n]

名 下顎前突症

> <u>下顎前突症</u>：顔面骨格に対して下顎骨が異常に前突していること．

2. 不正咬合

34. <u>bimaxillary protrusion</u>： The excessive forward projection of both the maxilla and the mandible in relation to the cranial base.

106 <u>bimaxillary protrusion</u>
[baimǽksəlèri proutrúːʒ(ə)n]

名 上下顎前突

107 <u>cranial</u>
[kréiniəl]

形 頭蓋の ← cranium (837)

108 <u>cranial base</u>
[kréiniəl béis]

名 頭蓋底

<u>上下顎前突</u>：頭蓋底に対して上顎骨・下顎骨双方が過度に前突していること．

---

35. <u>mandibular retrusion</u>： An abnormal posterior positioning of the mandible relative to the facial skeleton.

109 <u>mandibular retrusion</u>
[mændíbjələr ritrúːʒ(ə)n]

名 下顎後退症

110 <u>posterior</u>
[poustíəriər]

形 後方の ↔ anterior (89)

<u>下顎後退症</u>：顔面骨格に対して下顎骨が異常に後退していること．

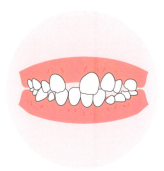

3 歯の硬組織疾患

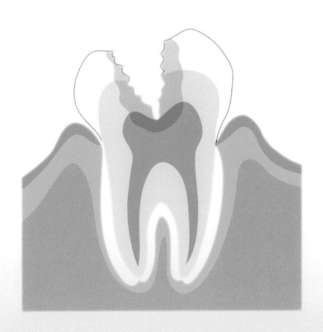

3. 歯の硬組織疾患

36. <u>dental caries</u> (=<u>tooth decay</u>): Localized, progressively destructive tooth disease that starts at the enamel with the dissolution of the inorganic components by organic acids that are produced in immediate proximity to the tooth by the enzymatic action of microorganisms on carbohydrates.

111 □ **dental caries** [dént(ə)l kéəriz] — 名 う蝕

112 □ **tooth decay** [túːθ dikéi] — 名 う蝕

113 □ **localized** [lóuk(ə)làizd] — 形 限局性の ↔ generalized (840)

114 □ **dissolution** [dìsəlúːʃ(ə)n] — 名 溶解

115 □ **inorganic** [ìnɔːrgǽnik] — 形 無機の

116 □ **organic** [ɔːrgǽnik] — 形 有機の

117 □ **organic acid** [ɔːrgǽnik ǽsəd] — 名 有機酸

118 □ **acid** [ǽsəd] — 名 酸

119 □ **enzymatic** [ènzəmǽtik] — 形 酵素の

120 □ **microorganism** [màikrouɔːrgənizm] — 名 微生物

121 □ **carbohydrate** [kàːrbouháidrèit] — 名 炭水化物

> う蝕：歯の限局性，進行性，破壊性疾患．エナメル質から始まり，炭水化物に対する微生物の酵素作用により歯の近接部で産生される有機酸による無機成分の溶解をともなう．

3. 歯の硬組織疾患

37. attrition: A type of tooth wear caused by tooth-to-tooth contact, resulting in loss of tooth structure, usually starting at the incisal edges or occlusal surfaces.

122 attrition
[ətríʃ(ə)n]

名 咬耗症

123 occlusal surface
[əklúːs(ə)l sə́ːrfəs]

名 咬合面

> **咬耗症**：歯の摩耗の一形態で歯と歯の接触に起因する．通常，切縁または咬合面から始まり，歯組織の欠損を生じる．

38. abrasion: Loss of tooth structure by mechanical forces from a foreign element, such as a toothbrush, a toothpick, or dental floss.

124 abrasion
[əbréiʒ(ə)n]

名 摩耗症

125 toothbrush
[túːθbrʌʃ]

名 歯ブラシ

126 toothpick
[túːθpik]

名 つま楊枝

127 dental floss
[dént(ə)l flɑ́s]

名 デンタルフロス

> **摩耗症**：歯ブラシ，つま楊枝，デンタルフロス等の外的要因からの物理的な力による歯組織の欠損．

39. erosion: Loss of tooth structure due to acids, such as carbonated beverages, citrus fruits, or stomach acid.

128 erosion
[iróuʒ(ə)n]

名 酸蝕症

129 stomach acid
[stʌ́mək ǽsəd]

名 胃酸

> **酸蝕症**：炭酸飲料，柑橘類，胃酸等の酸による歯組織の欠損．

3．歯の硬組織疾患

40. abfraction：Loss of tooth structure caused by excessive occlusal forces such as bruxism and added abrasive components such as a toothbrush and toothpaste.

130 □ abfraction
[æbfrǽkʃ(ə)n]
名 アブフラクション

131 □ occlusal force
[əklúːs(ə)l fɔ́ːrs]
名 咬合力

132 □ bruxism
[brʌ́ksìzm]
名 歯ぎしり

133 □ toothpaste
[túːθpèist]
名 練り歯磨き

> **アブフラクション**：歯ぎしり等の過度な咬合力に歯ブラシや練り歯磨き等の摩耗要因が加わることで引き起こされる歯組織の欠損．

41. wedge-shaped defect：Wedge-shaped abfraction lesions located along the gingival margin.

134 □ wedge-shaped defect
[wédʒ ʃéipt díːfèkt]
名 くさび状欠損

135 □ lesion
[líːʒ(ə)n]
名 病変

136 □ gingival
[dʒíndʒəv(ə)l]
形 歯肉の ← gingiva (167)

137 □ gingival margin
[dʒíndʒəv(ə)l máːrdʒən]
名 歯肉縁

> **くさび状欠損**：歯肉縁沿いに見られるくさび状のアブフラクション病変．

3. 歯の硬組織疾患

42. fracture : The cracking or breaking of a tooth.

138 fracture
[fræktʃər]

名 破折

破折：歯が割れる，または折れること．

43. luxation : The dislocation or displacement of a tooth from the alveolus.

139 luxation
[lʌkséiʃ(ə)n]

名 脱臼

140 alveolus
[ælvíːələs]

名 歯槽

脱臼：歯槽からの歯の変位または脱離．

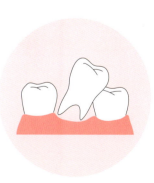

4 歯髄・歯周組織疾患

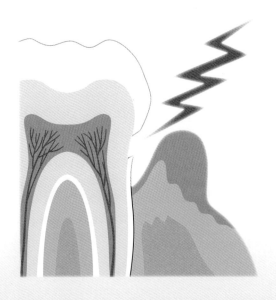

4. 歯髄・歯周組織疾患

44. dentin hypersensitivity: Transient painful reaction that occurs when some areas of exposed dentin are subjected to a mechanical, thermal, or chemical stimulus.

141 □ **dentin hypersensitivity**
[déntən hàipərsènsətívəti]
名 象牙質知覚過敏症

142 □ **hypersensitivity**
[hàipərsènsətívəti]
名 過敏症

> 象牙質知覚過敏症：露出した象牙質面が物理的, 温度的, 化学的刺激を受けた際に生じる一過性の疼痛反応.

45. denticle (=pulp stone): A calcified body found in the pulp cavity of a tooth having dentin-like structure.

143 □ **denticle**
[déntikl]
名 象牙質粒

144 □ **pulp stone**
[pʌ́lp stóun]
名 歯髄結石

145 □ **calcified**
[kǽlsəfàid]
形 石灰化した → calcification (327)

> 象牙質粒(= 歯髄結石)：歯髄腔内に形成される象牙質様の構造をもつ石灰化小体.

46. pulp hyperemia: An increased amount of blood flow in the dental pulp resulting in vascular congestion.

146 □ **pulp hyperemia**
[pʌ́lp hàipərí:miə]
名 歯髄充血

147 □ **hyperemia**
[hàipərí:miə]
名 充血

148 □ **dental pulp**
[dént(ə)l pʌ́lp]
名 歯髄

149 □ **vascular**
[vǽskjələr]
形 血管の

150 □ **congestion**
[kəndʒést∫(ə)n]
名 うっ血

> 歯髄充血：歯髄における血流量の増加で, 血管のうっ血を生じる.

4. 歯髄・歯周組織疾患

47. pulpitis: Inflammation of the dental pulp resulting from dental caries or trauma.

151 **pulpitis** [pÀlpáitəs] — 名 歯髄炎

> 歯髄炎：う蝕または外傷に起因する歯髄の炎症．

48. pulp necrosis: Death of pulp tissue due to chronic pulpitis or to trauma and subsequent occlusion of the apical blood vessel.

152 **pulp necrosis** [pÁlp nekróusəs] — 名 歯髄壊死

153 **necrosis** [nekróusəs] — 名 壊死

154 **chronic** [kránik] — 形 慢性の ↔ acute (181)

155 **chronic pulpitis** [kránik pÀlpáitəs] — 名 慢性歯髄炎

156 **occlusion** [əklúːʒ(ə)n] — 名 閉塞

157 **apical** [ǽpik(ə)l] — 形 根尖(部)の

158 **blood vessel** [blÁd vés(ə)l] — 名 血管

> 歯髄壊死：慢性歯髄炎または外傷にともなう根尖部血管の閉塞に起因する歯髄組織の死．

49. root resorption: Dissolution of the root of a tooth; either external resorption with loss of cementum from the outside, or internal resorption with loss of dentin from the inside.

159 **root resorption** [rúːt risɔ́ːrpʃ(ə)n] — 名 歯根吸収

160 **external resorption** [ikstə́ːrn(ə)l risɔ́ːrpʃ(ə)n] — 名 外部吸収

161 **internal resorption** [intə́ːrn(ə)l risɔ́ːrpʃ(ə)n] — 名 内部吸収

4. 歯髄・歯周組織疾患

> **歯根吸収**：歯根の溶解．外側からセメント質が欠けていく外部吸収と，内側から象牙質が欠けていく内部吸収とがある．

50. apical periodontitis：Inflammation of the periodontal tissue around the root apex of a tooth.

162 apical periodontitis
[ǽpik(ə)l pèrioudòntáitəs]
名 根尖性歯周炎

163 periodontitis
[pèrioudòntáitəs]
名 歯周炎

164 periodontal
[pèrioudónt(ə)l]
形 歯周の

165 root apex
[rúːt éipèks]
名 根尖

> **根尖性歯周炎**：歯の根尖周囲の歯周組織の炎症．

51. gingivitis：Inflammation of the gingiva as a response to dental plaque on adjacent teeth, characterized by redness, swelling, and bleeding.

166 gingivitis
[dʒindʒəváitəs]
名 歯肉炎

167 gingiva
[dʒíndʒəvə]
名 歯肉

168 dental plaque
[dént(ə)l plǽk]
名 歯垢，プラーク

169 redness
[rédnəs]
名 発赤

170 swelling
[swéliŋ]
名 腫脹

171 bleeding
[blíːdiŋ]
名 出血 = hemorrhage (371)

> **歯肉炎**：隣接する歯の歯垢に反応して生じる歯肉の炎症．発赤，腫脹，出血等を特徴とする．

4. 歯髄・歯周組織疾患

52. desquamative gingivitis: Inflammation of the gingiva usually occurring in middle-aged women and characterized by pain, erythema, mucosal atrophy, and desquamation.

172 ☐ desquamative gingivitis [diskwǽmətiv dʒìndʒəváitəs] — 名 剥離性歯肉炎

173 ☐ pain [péin] — 名 疼痛

174 ☐ erythema [èrəθíːmə] — 名 紅斑

175 ☐ mucosal [mjukóus(ə)l] — 形 粘膜の ← mucosa (194)

176 ☐ atrophy [ǽtrəfi] — 名 萎縮

177 ☐ desquamation [dèskwəméiʃ(ə)n] — 名 剥離

剥離性歯肉炎：中年の女性に好発し，疼痛，紅斑，粘膜の萎縮，剥離等を特徴とする歯肉の炎症．

53. necrotizing ulcerative gingivitis: An acute gingivitis characterized by gingival erythema and pain, halitosis, necrosis, and sloughing of interdental papillae and marginal gingiva.

178 ☐ necrotizing ulcerative gingivitis [nékrətàiziŋ ʌ́lsərətiv dʒìndʒəváitəs] — 名 壊死性潰瘍性歯肉炎

179 ☐ necrotizing [nékrətàiziŋ] — 形 壊死性の ← necrosis (153)

180 ☐ ulcerative [ʌ́lsərətiv] — 形 潰瘍(性)の ← ulcer (538)

181 ☐ acute [əkjúːt] — 形 急性の ↔ chronic (154)

182 ☐ halitosis [hæ̀lətóusəs] — 名 口臭

183 ☐ slough [slʌ́f] — 動 (壊死部分が)脱落する

4. 歯髄・歯周組織疾患

184 ☐ **interdental papillae**
[ìntərdént(ə)l pəpíli:]

名 **歯間乳頭**（複；単〜 papilla [pəpílə]）

185 ☐ **papilla**
[pəpílə]

名 **乳頭**（複 papillae [pəpíli:]）

186 ☐ **marginal gingiva**
[má:rdʒən(ə)l dʒíndʒəvə]

名 **辺縁歯肉**

> **壊死性潰瘍性歯肉炎**：歯肉の紅斑と疼痛，口臭，壊死，歯間乳頭および辺縁歯肉の脱落等を特徴とする急性の歯肉炎．

54. gingival abscess : A collection of pus localized in the gingival soft tissue.

187 ☐ **gingival abscess**
[dʒíndʒəv(ə)l ǽbsès]

名 **歯肉膿瘍**

188 ☐ **abscess**
[ǽbsès]

名 **膿瘍**

189 ☐ **pus**
[pʌs]

名 **膿**

190 ☐ **soft tissue**
[sɔ́ft tíʃu]

名 **軟組織**

> **歯肉膿瘍**：歯肉の軟組織に限局した膿の蓄積．

55. dental fistula : An abnormal passage from the apical periodontal area of a tooth to the surface of the oral mucosa, permitting the discharge of suppurative material.

191 ☐ **dental fistula**
[dént(ə)l fístʃələ]

名 **歯瘻**

192 ☐ **fistula**
[fístʃələ]

名 **瘻孔**

193 ☐ **oral mucosa**
[ɔ́:r(ə)l mjukóusə]

名 **口腔粘膜**

4. 歯髄・歯周組織疾患

194 mucosa
[mjukóusə]

名 粘膜 = mucous membrane (569)

195 suppurative
[sápjərèitiv]

形 化膿性の

> 歯瘻：歯の根尖歯周部から口腔粘膜表面へ通じる異常な通路で，化膿性物質を排出する．

56. chronic periodontitis：Chronic inflammation of the periodontium due to accumulation of dental plaque and calculus, characterized by gingivitis, periodontal pocket formation, and destruction of alveolar bone and periodontal ligament.

196 chronic periodontitis
[kránik pèrioudùntáitəs]

名 慢性歯周炎

197 periodontium
[pèrioudánʃ(i)əm]

名 歯周組織

198 dental calculus
[dént(ə)l kǽlkjələs]

名 歯石 = tartar (988)

199 periodontal pocket
[pèrioudánt(ə)l pákət]

名 歯周ポケット

200 alveolar
[ælvíːələr]

形 歯槽の ← alveolus (140)

201 alveolar bone
[ælvíːələr bóun]

名 歯槽骨

202 periodontal ligament
[pèrioudánt(ə)l lígəmənt]

名 歯周靱帯 = periodontal membrane (342)

203 ligament
[lígəmənt]

名 靱帯

> 慢性歯周炎：歯垢および歯石の蓄積に起因する慢性の歯周組織の炎症で，歯肉炎，歯周ポケットの形成，歯槽骨や歯周靱帯の破壊等を特徴とする．

4．歯髄・歯周組織疾患

57. occlusal trauma：Injury to a tooth and surrounding structures caused by occlusal forces.

204 □ occlusal trauma
[əklúːs(ə)l trɔ́ːmə]

205 □ injury
[índʒəri]

名 咬合性外傷

名 損傷，外傷

咬合性外傷：咬合力に起因する歯および周辺組織の損傷．

58. gingival recession：The drawing back of the gingiva from the necks of the teeth, with exposure of root surfaces.

206 □ gingival recession
[dʒíndʒəv(ə)l riséʃ(ə)n]

207 □ neck of tooth
[nék əv túːθ]

名 歯肉退縮

名 歯頸部

歯肉退縮：歯頸部から歯肉が後退し，歯根表面が露出すること．

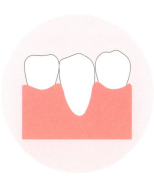

5 顎・口腔領域の先天異常と変形

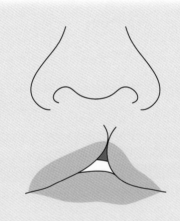

5. 顎・口腔領域の先天異常と変形

59. <u>cleft lip</u> : A congenital fissure of the lip resulting from incomplete fusion of the medial nasal process and the maxillary process during embryonic development.

208 ☐ <u>cleft lip</u>
[kléft líp]
名 口唇裂

209 ☐ fissure
[fíʃər]
名 裂

210 ☐ medial
[míːdiəl]
形 内側の ↔ lateral (30)

211 ☐ nasal process
[néiz(ə)l prásès]
名 鼻突起

212 ☐ maxillary process
[mǽksəlèri prásès]
名 上顎突起

213 ☐ embryonic
[èmbriánik]
形 胚の

<u>口唇裂</u>：口唇の先天性の裂で，胚発生期における内側鼻突起と上顎突起の融合不全から生じる．

---

60. <u>alveolar cleft</u> : A congenital fissure in the alveolar process that typically occurs with a cleft lip.

214 ☐ <u>alveolar cleft</u>
[ælvíːələr kléft]
名 歯槽裂，顎裂

215 ☐ alveolar process
[ælvíːələr prásès]
名 歯槽突起

<u>歯槽裂（= 顎裂）</u>：通常，口唇裂にともなって生じる歯槽突起の先天性の裂．

---

61. <u>cleft palate</u> : A congenital fissure in the superior wall of the oral cavity resulting from incomplete fusion of the palatine processes.

216 ☐ <u>cleft palate</u>
[kléft pǽlət]
名 口蓋裂

217 ☐ palate
[pǽlət]
名 口蓋

218 ☐ superior
[supíəriər]
形 上部の，上方の ↔ inferior (359)

5. 顎・口腔領域の先天異常と変形

219 oral cavity
[ɔ́ːr(ə)l kǽvəti]

名 口腔

220 palatine process
[pǽlətàin prɑ́sès]

名 口蓋突起

> 口蓋裂：口腔上壁の先天性の裂で，口蓋突起の融合不全から生じる．

62. facial cleft : A collective term for all sorts of congenital gaps in the face, such as median facial cleft, transverse facial cleft, and oblique facial cleft.

221 facial cleft
[féiʃ(ə)l kléft]

名 顔面裂

222 median
[míːdiən]

形 正中の

223 median facial cleft
[míːdiən féiʃ(ə)l kléft]

名 正中顔面裂

224 transverse facial cleft
[trænsvə́ːrs féiʃ(ə)l kléft]

名 横顔（面）裂

225 oblique facial cleft
[əblíːk féiʃ(ə)l kléft]

名 斜顔（面）裂

> 顔面裂：顔面における先天性の裂の総称で，正中顔面裂，横顔（面）裂，斜顔（面）裂等を含む．

63. submucous cleft palate : A separation of the bone in the hard palate or muscle in the soft palate, but with full closure of the overlying mucosa.

226 submucous cleft palate
[sʌ̀bmjúːkəs kléft pǽlət]

名 粘膜下口蓋裂

227 submucous
[sʌ̀bmjúːkəs]

形 粘膜下の

228 hard palate
[hɑ́ːrd pǽlət]

名 硬口蓋

229 muscle
[mʌ́s(ə)l]

名 筋

230 soft palate
[sɔ́ft pǽlət]

名 軟口蓋

> 粘膜下口蓋裂：硬口蓋の骨や軟口蓋の筋に裂が見られるが，上を覆う粘膜は完全に結合している状態．

5. 顎・口腔領域の先天異常と変形

64. congenital velopharyngeal insufficiency: A congenital defect of the soft palate or superior pharyngeal constrictor muscle, resulting in the inability to achieve velopharyngeal closure.

231 congenital velopharyngeal insufficiency
[kəndʒénit(ə)l vìːloufæ̀rəndʒíːəl ìnsəfíʃənsi]
名 先天性鼻咽腔閉鎖不全症

232 velopharyngeal
[vìːloufæ̀rəndʒíːəl]
形 口蓋咽頭の

233 superior pharyngeal constrictor muscle
[supíəriər fæ̀rəndʒíːəl kənstríktər mʌ́s(ə)l]
名 上咽頭収縮筋

先天性鼻咽腔閉鎖不全症：軟口蓋または上咽頭収縮筋の先天性欠陥で，口蓋咽頭の閉鎖不全を生じる．

65. macrocheilia: Abnormally enlarged lips resulting from lip sucking habit, hypothyroidism, hemangioma, or lymphangioma.

234 macrocheilia
[mæ̀kroukáiliə]
名 巨唇症

235 lip sucking habit
[líp sʌ́kiŋ hǽbət]
名 吸唇癖

236 hypothyroidism
[hàipouθáiərɔidìzm]
名 甲状腺機能低下症

237 hemangioma
[hìːmændʒióumə]
名 血管腫

238 lymphangioma
[lìmfændʒióumə]
名 リンパ管腫

巨唇症：吸唇癖，甲状腺機能低下症，血管腫，リンパ管腫等に起因する口唇の異常な肥大．

5. 顎・口腔領域の先天異常と変形

66. double lip：Congenital or acquired fold of excess tissue on the mucosal surface of the upper lip.

239 □ double lip
[dʎbl líp]

240 □ acquired
[əkwáiərd]

名 二重唇

形 後天的な，後天性の ↔ congenital (9)

二重唇：上唇の粘膜表面における先天性または後天性のヒダ状の過剰組織．

67. microstomia：A congenital or acquired reduction in the size of the oral aperture.

241 □ microstomia
[màikroustóumiə]

242 □ aperture
[ǽpərtʃər]

名 小口症

名 開口部

小口症：先天的または後天的に口の開口部が小さいこと．

68. masseter muscle hypertrophy：Unilateral or bilateral chronic enlargement of the masseter muscles.

243 □ masseter muscle hypertrophy
[mæsí:tər mʎs(ə)l haipə́:rtrəfi]

244 □ masseter muscle
[mæsí:tər mʎs(ə)l]

245 □ hypertrophy
[haipə́:rtrəfi]

246 □ unilateral
[jù:nəlǽtər(ə)l]

247 □ bilateral
[bailǽtər(ə)l]

名 咬筋肥大症

名 咬筋

名 肥大

形 片側の

形 両側の

咬筋肥大症：片側または両側の咬筋の慢性的肥大．

5. 顎・口腔領域の先天異常と変形

69. macroglossia：Enlargement of the tongue, either congenital in origin or secondary to edema, tumors, endocrine disturbance, or accumulation of substances.

248 □ **macroglossia**
[mæ̀krouglásiə]
名 巨舌症

249 □ **edema**
[idíːmə]
名 浮腫

250 □ **tumor**
[t(j)úːmər]
名 腫瘍

251 □ **endocrine**
[éndəkrən]
形 内分泌の

<u>巨舌症</u>：先天性の原因，もしくは浮腫，腫瘍，内分泌障害，物質の蓄積等にともなう舌の肥大．

70. microglossia：A rare congenital malformation characterized by an abnormally small tongue.

252 □ **microglossia**
[màikrouglásiə]
名 小舌症

<u>小舌症</u>：異常に小さな舌を特徴とするまれな先天性奇形．

71. cleft tongue：A congenital malformation of the tongue in which its anterior part is divided longitudinally.

253 □ **cleft tongue**
[kléft tʌ́ŋ]
名 舌裂

<u>舌裂</u>：舌の先天性の奇形で，前部が縦に分裂している．

72. lingual thyroid：A nodule of ectopic thyroid tissue located at the base of the tongue.

254 □ **lingual thyroid**
[líŋwəl θáiərɔ̀id]
名 舌甲状腺

255 □ **thyroid**
[θáiərɔ̀id]
名 甲状腺　形 甲状腺の

5. 顎・口腔領域の先天異常と変形

256 ectopic
[ektápik]

形 異所性の

舌甲状腺：舌底部に見られる異所性甲状腺組織の小結節．

73. epithelial pearls : Multiple nodules in the gingiva of neonates, derived from remnants of the dental lamina.

257 epithelial pearls
[èpəθíːliəl páːrlz]

名 上皮真珠

258 epithelial
[èpəθíːliəl]

形 上皮(性)の ← epithelium (334)

259 multiple
[máltəp(ə)l]

形 多発性の

260 neonate
[níːənèit]

名 新生児

261 remnant
[rémnənt]

名 遺残組織

262 dental lamina
[dént(ə)l lǽmənə]

名 歯堤

上皮真珠：新生児の歯肉に生じる多発性の小結節．歯堤の遺残組織に由来する．

74. gingival fibromatosis : A noninflammatory condition characterized by fibrous hyperplasia of the gingiva.

263 gingival fibromatosis
[dʒíndʒəv(ə)l faibròumətóusəs]

名 歯肉線維腫症

264 fibromatosis
[faibròumətóusəs]

名 線維腫症 ← fibroma (433)

265 noninflammatory
[nùninflǽmətɔ̀ːri]

形 非炎症性の

266 fibrous
[fáibrəs]

形 線維性の

267 hyperplasia
[hàipərpléiʒ(i)ə]

名 増殖，過形成

5. 顎・口腔領域の先天異常と変形

> <u>歯肉線維腫症</u>：歯肉の線維性増殖を特徴とする非炎症性疾患．

75. gingival hyperplasia：Diffuse enlargement of the gingiva due to hereditary or metabolic disorders, or drugs such as phenytoin, cyclosporine, and nifedipine.

268 □ **gingival hyperplasia**
[dʒíndʒəv(ə)l hàipərpléiʒ(i)ə]
名 歯肉増殖

269 □ **diffuse**
[difjúːs]
形 びまん性の

270 □ **hereditary**
[hərédətèri]
形 遺伝性の ← heredity (989)

271 □ **metabolic**
[mètəbálik]
形 代謝性の ← metabolism (744)

272 □ **phenytoin**
[fənítouən]
名 フェニトイン（抗痙攣薬）

273 □ **cyclosporine**
[sàikləspóːrən]
名 シクロスポリン（免疫抑制薬）

274 □ **nifedipine**
[naifédəpìːn]
名 ニフェジピン（血圧降下薬）

> <u>歯肉増殖</u>：遺伝性疾患，代謝性疾患，またはフェニトイン，シクロスポリン，ニフェジピン等の薬物に起因する歯肉のびまん性肥大．

76. high-arched palate：An unusually high palate that may occur in association with a number of hereditary disorders of the skeletal system.

275 □ **high-arched palate**
[hái áːrtʃt pælət]
名 高口蓋

276 □ **skeletal**
[skélət(ə)l]
形 骨格の ← skeleton (104)

277 □ **skeletal system**
[skélət(ə)l sístəm]
名 骨格系

> <u>高口蓋</u>：さまざまな遺伝性の骨格系疾患にともなって見られる異常に高い口蓋．

5. 顎・口腔領域の先天異常と変形

77. ankyloglossia: A congenital malformation in which a short lingual frenulum restricts tongue movement.

278 □ **ankyloglossia**
[æ̀ŋkəlouglásiə]

名 舌小帯短縮症

279 □ **lingual frenulum**
[líŋwəl frénjələm]

名 舌小帯

280 □ **frenulum**
[frénjələm]

名 小帯

> **舌小帯短縮症**：短い舌小帯により舌の動きが制限される先天性奇形．

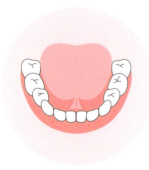

6 軟組織の炎症

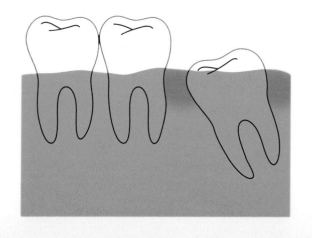

6. 軟組織の炎症

78. pericoronitis: Acute or chronic inflammation of the gingiva around the crown of an incompletely erupted tooth, usually the third molar.

281 □ **pericoronitis**
[pèrikɔ̀:rənáitəs]

名 歯冠周囲炎，智歯周囲炎

282 □ **third molar**
[θə́:rd móulər]

名 第三大臼歯

歯冠周囲炎（= 智歯周囲炎）：不完全萌出歯（通常は第三大臼歯）の歯冠周囲の歯肉の急性または慢性の炎症．

79. cellulitis: A diffuse suppurative inflammation of the skin and subcutaneous tissue.

283 □ **cellulitis**
[sèljəláitəs]

名 蜂窩織炎，蜂巣炎

284 □ **skin**
[skín]

名 皮膚

285 □ **subcutaneous**
[sʌ̀bkjutéiniəs]

形 皮下の

286 □ **subcutaneous tissue**
[sʌ̀bkjutéiniəs tíʃu]

名 皮下組織

蜂窩織炎（= 蜂巣炎）：皮膚および皮下組織のびまん性の化膿性炎症．

80. Ludwig's angina: A severe form of cellulitis of the submaxillary space and secondary involvement of the sublingual and submental spaces, usually resulting from an infection in the mandibular molar area or a penetrating injury of the floor of the mouth.

287 □ **Ludwig's angina**
[lú:dvigz ændʒáinə]

名 ルートヴィヒアンギナ

288 □ **angina**
[ændʒáinə]

名 アンギナ

289 □ **submaxillary**
[sʌ̀bmæksəlèri]

形 下顎の

6. 軟組織の炎症

290 **sublingual** [sÀblíŋwəl]	形 舌下の
291 **submental** [sÀbmént(ə)l]	形 オトガイ下の ← mental (990)
292 **infection** [infékʃ(ə)n]	名 感染，感染症
293 **floor of mouth** [flɔ́ːr əv máuθ]	名 口底

> **ルートヴィヒアンギナ**：下顎隙の蜂窩織炎の重症型で，舌下隙およびオトガイ下隙への2次的侵襲をともなう．通常，下顎大臼歯部の感染症または口底の穿通性損傷に起因する．

81. odontogenic peritonsillitis：Inflammation of the connective tissue surrounding the tonsils associated with pericoronitis or infection after wisdom tooth extraction.

294 **odontogenic peritonsillitis** [oudàntoudʒénik pèritànsəláitəs]	名 歯性扁桃周囲炎
295 **odontogenic** [oudàntoudʒénik]	形 歯(性)の
296 **peritonsillitis** [pèritànsəláitəs]	名 扁桃周囲炎 ← tonsillitis (991)
297 **connective tissue** [kənéktiv tíʃu]	名 結合組織
298 **tonsil** [táns(ə)l]	名 扁桃
299 **wisdom tooth** [wízdəm túːθ]	名 智歯
300 **extraction** [ikstrǽkʃ(ə)n]	名 抜歯

> **歯性扁桃周囲炎**：歯冠周囲炎や智歯の抜歯後感染に関連する扁桃周囲の結合組織の炎症．

6. 軟組織の炎症

82. odontogenic maxillary sinusitis: Suppurative inflammation of the maxillary sinus associated with apical or marginal periodontitis.

301 □ odontogenic maxillary sinusitis
[oudàntoudʒénik mæksəlèri sàinəsáitəs]

|名| 歯性上顎洞炎

302 □ sinusitis
[sàinəsáitəs]

|名| 副鼻腔炎

303 □ maxillary sinus
[mǽksəlèri sáinəs]

|名| 上顎洞

304 □ marginal periodontitis
[máːrdʒən(ə)l pèrioudʌ̀ntáitəs]

|名| 辺縁性歯周炎

<u>歯性上顎洞炎</u>：根尖性歯周炎や辺縁性歯周炎に関連する上顎洞の化膿性炎症．

---

83. actinomycosis: A chronic infection caused by *Actinomyces* and characterized by a local abscess with draining sinuses and low-grade septicemia.

305 □ actinomycosis
[æktənoumaikóusəs]

|名| 放線菌症

306 □ *Actinomyces*
[æktənoumáisìːz]

|名| 放線菌属

307 □ draining sinus
[dréiniŋ sáinəs]

|名| 排膿瘻孔

308 □ septicemia
[sèptəsíːmiə]

|名| 敗血症

<u>放線菌症</u>：放線菌属による慢性の感染症で，排膿瘻孔をともなう局所の膿瘍と軽度の敗血症を特徴とする．

6. 軟組織の炎症

84. <u>lupus vulgaris</u>: Cutaneous tuberculosis with characteristic nodular lesions on the face, particularly about the nose and ears.

309 □ <u>lupus vulgaris</u>　　　　　名 尋常性狼瘡
[lú:pəs vàlgǽrəs]

310 □ lupus　　　　　　　　　名 狼瘡
[lú:pəs]

311 □ cutaneous　　　　　　　形 皮膚の
[kjutéiniəs]

312 □ tuberculosis　　　　　　名 結核
[t(j)ubə̀:rkjəlóusəs]

313 □ nodular　　　　　　　　形 小結節性の ← nodule (46)
[nádʒələr]

<u>尋常性狼瘡</u>：顔面，とくに鼻および耳の周囲の特徴的な小結節性病変をともなう皮膚結核．

85. <u>tuberculous cervical lymphadenitis</u>: Tuberculosis of cervical lymph nodes, with granuloma formation and caseous necrosis.

314 □ <u>tuberculous cervical lymphadenitis</u>　　名 結核性頸部リンパ節炎
[t(j)ubə́:rkjələs sə́:rvik(ə)l lìmfædənáitəs]

315 □ tuberculous　　　　　　形 結核(性)の ← tuberculosis (312)
[t(j)ubə́:rkjələs]

316 □ lymphadenitis　　　　　名 リンパ節炎
[lìmfædənáitəs]

317 □ lymph node　　　　　　名 リンパ節
[límf nóud]

318 □ granuloma　　　　　　　名 肉芽腫
[græ̀njəlóumə]

319 □ caseous　　　　　　　　形 乾酪性の
[kéisiəs]

320 □ caseous necrosis　　　　名 乾酪壊死
[kéisiəs nekróusəs]

<u>結核性頸部リンパ節炎</u>：肉芽腫形成と乾酪壊死をともなう頸部リンパ節の結核．

7 | 囊胞性疾患

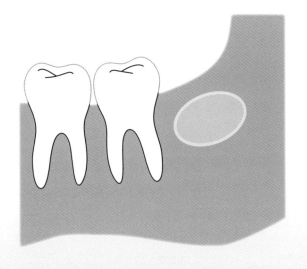

7. 囊胞性疾患

86. <u>primordial cyst</u>: An odontogenic cyst that develops through cystic degeneration of the enamel organ before calcification.

321 <u>primordial cyst</u> [praimɔ́ːrdiəl síst]	名 原始性囊胞
322 cyst [síst]	名 囊胞
323 odontogenic cyst [oudàntoudʒénik síst]	名 歯原性囊胞
324 cystic [sístik]	形 囊胞の，囊胞性の ← cyst (322)
325 degeneration [didʒènəréiʃ(ə)n]	名 変性
326 enamel organ [inǽm(ə)l ɔ́ːrgən]	名 エナメル器
327 calcification [kæ̀lsəfəkéiʃ(ə)n]	名 石灰化

<u>原始性囊胞</u>：エナメル器が石灰化前に囊胞変性を起こすことにより生じる歯原性囊胞.

87. <u>odontogenic keratocyst</u>: A cyst of dental lamina origin lined with layers of orthokeratinized stratified squamous epithelium that most often affects the posterior mandible.

328 <u>odontogenic keratocyst</u> [oudàntoudʒénik kérətousìst]	名 歯原性角化囊胞
329 keratocyst [kérətousìst]	名 角化囊胞
330 line [láin]	動 裏装する
331 orthokeratinized [ɔ̀ːrθoukérətənàizd]	形 正角化の ← keratinized (404)
332 stratified squamous epithelium [strǽtəfàid skwéiməs èpəθíːliəm]	名 重層扁平上皮
333 squamous epithelium [skwéiməs èpəθíːliəm]	名 扁平上皮

7. 囊胞性疾患

334 epithelium
[èpəθíːliəm]

名 上皮

歯原性角化囊胞：数層の正角化重層扁平上皮で裏装された歯堤由来の囊胞で，下顎の後方部に好発する．

88. dentigerous cyst (=follicular dental cyst)：An odontogenic cyst derived from the reduced enamel epithelium, surrounding the crown of an impacted tooth.

335 dentigerous cyst
[dentídʒərəs síst]

名 含歯性囊胞

336 follicular dental cyst
[fəlíkjələr dént(ə)l síst]

名 濾胞性歯囊胞

337 follicular
[fəlíkjələr]

形 濾胞性の，小胞性の

338 enamel epithelium
[inǽm(ə)l èpəθíːliəm]

名 エナメル上皮

含歯性囊胞（= 濾胞性歯囊胞）：退縮エナメル上皮に由来し，埋伏歯の歯冠を覆う歯原性囊胞．

89. eruption cyst：A form of dentigerous cyst that occurs on the alveolar mucosa over an erupting tooth.

339 eruption cyst
[irʌ́pʃ(ə)n síst]

名 萌出囊胞

340 alveolar mucosa
[ælvíːələr mjukóusə]

名 歯槽粘膜

萌出囊胞：萌出中の歯を覆う歯槽粘膜に生じる含歯性囊胞の一種．

7. 囊胞性疾患

90. lateral periodontal cyst: A cyst derived from remnants of odontogenic epithelium that occurs on the periodontal membrane of an erupted vital tooth.

341 □ lateral periodontal cyst
[lǽtər(ə)l pèrioudánt(ə)l síst]
名 側方性歯周囊胞

342 □ periodontal membrane
[pèrioudánt(ə)l mémbrèin]
名 歯根膜 = periodontal ligament (202)

343 □ membrane
[mémbrèin]
名 膜

344 □ vital tooth
[váit(ə)l tú:θ]
名 生活歯 ↔ nonvital tooth (366)

> **側方性歯周囊胞**：歯原性上皮の遺残組織に由来する囊胞で，萌出した生活歯の歯根膜に生じる．

91. gingival cyst: A small cyst occurring in either the free gingiva or attached gingiva, most frequently seen near mandibular canine and premolar region.

345 □ gingival cyst
[dʒíndʒəv(ə)l síst]
名 歯肉囊胞

346 □ free gingiva
[frí: dʒíndʒəvə]
名 遊離歯肉

347 □ attached gingiva
[ətǽtʃt dʒíndʒəvə]
名 付着歯肉

348 □ canine
[kéinàin]
名 犬歯 = cuspid (992)

349 □ premolar
[prì:móulər]
名 小臼歯

> **歯肉囊胞**：遊離歯肉または付着歯肉に生じる小囊胞で，下顎犬歯および小臼歯部に好発する．

92. glandular odontogenic cyst: A rare cyst occurring mainly in middle-aged people with the anterior mandible as the common site of occurrence, which may appear as a unilocular or multilocular lesion in radiographs.

350 □ glandular odontogenic cyst
[glǽndʒələr oudàntoudʒénik síst]
名 腺性歯原性囊胞

7. 囊胞性疾患

351 □ **glandular**
[glǽndʒələr]

形 腺(性)の ← gland (385)

352 □ **unilocular**
[jùːnəlákjələr]

形 単房性の

353 □ **multilocular**
[mÀltilákjələr]

形 多房性の

354 □ **radiograph**
[réidiougrǽf]

名 エックス線写真

> **腺性歯原性囊胞**：主に中年期の人びとに見られる下顎骨前部を好発部位とするまれな囊胞．エックス線写真では単房性または多房性の病変像を呈する．

93. <u>nasopalatine duct cyst</u>：A cyst in or near the incisive canal, derived from epithelial remnants of the nasopalatine duct.

355 □ **nasopalatine duct cyst**
[nèizoupǽlətàin dÁkt síst]

名 鼻口蓋管囊胞

356 □ **nasopalatine duct**
[nèizoupǽlətàin dÁkt]

名 鼻口蓋管

357 □ **incisive canal**
[insáisiv kənǽl]

名 切歯管

> **鼻口蓋管囊胞**：切歯管の内部または近辺に生じる囊胞で，鼻口蓋管の上皮性遺残組織に由来する．

94. <u>nasoalveolar cyst</u>：A soft tissue cyst occurring inferior to the nasal ala, derived from epithelial remnants of the nasolacrimal duct.

358 □ **nasoalveolar cyst**
[nèizouælvíːələr síst]

名 鼻歯槽囊胞

359 □ **inferior**
[infíəriər]

形 下部の，下方の ↔ superior (218)

360 □ **nasal ala**
[néiz(ə)l éilə]

名 鼻翼

361 □ **nasolacrimal duct**
[nèizoulǽkrəml dÁkt]

名 鼻涙管

> **鼻歯槽囊胞**：鼻翼の下部の軟組織に生じる囊胞で，鼻涙管の上皮性遺残組織に由来する．

7. 囊胞性疾患

95. radicular cyst：An inflammatory odontogenic cyst occurring in the periapical region of a nonvital tooth.

362 ☐ **radicular cyst**
[rədíkjələr síst]

名 歯根嚢胞

363 ☐ **radicular**
[rədíkjələr]

形 歯根の

364 ☐ **inflammatory**
[inflǽmətɔ̀:ri]

形 炎症性の ← inflammation (62)

365 ☐ **periapical**
[pèriǽpik(ə)l]

形 根尖周囲の ← apical (157)

366 ☐ **nonvital tooth**
[nɑnváit(ə)l tú:θ]

名 失活歯 ↔ vital tooth (344)

歯根嚢胞：失活歯の根尖周囲に生じる炎症性の歯原性嚢胞.

---

96. residual cyst：A radicular cyst that remains after extraction of the offending tooth.

367 ☐ **residual cyst**
[rizídʒuəl síst]

名 残留嚢胞

残留嚢胞：原因歯の抜歯後も残存している歯根嚢胞.

---

97. paradental cyst：A cyst occurring near to the cervical margin of the lateral aspect of the roots as a consequence of inflammation in the periodontal pocket.

368 ☐ **paradental cyst**
[pæ̀rədént(ə)l síst]

名 歯周嚢胞

歯周嚢胞：歯周ポケット内の炎症の結果として歯根側面の歯頸縁付近に生じる嚢胞.

---

98. simple bone cyst：A benign empty lesion within bone which can result from hemorrhage caused by trauma, inadequate drainage of venous blood, or disturbance of local bone growth.

369 ☐ **simple bone cyst**
[símpl bóun síst]

名 単純性骨嚢胞

7. 囊胞性疾患

370 **benign** [bináin] 形 良性の ↔ malignant (458)

371 **hemorrhage** [héməridʒ] 名 出血 = bleeding (171)

372 **venous** [víːnəs] 形 静脈の

> 単純性骨囊胞：骨内に生じる良性の空洞状病変．外傷による出血，静脈血の不十分な排出，局所的な骨の発育異常等に起因する．

99. aneurysmal bone cyst：A solitary benign osteolytic lesion in a long bone or a vertebra, consisting of multilocular blood-filled spaces separated by fibrous tissue containing multinucleated giant cells.

373 **aneurysmal bone cyst** [ænjərízm(ə)l bóun síst] 名 脈瘤性骨囊胞

374 **aneurysmal** [ænjərízm(ə)l] 形 動脈瘤の ← aneurysm (993)

375 **solitary** [sálətèri] 形 孤立性の

376 **osteolytic** [àstiəlítik] 形 溶骨性の

377 **long bone** [lɔ́ŋ bóun] 名 長骨

378 **vertebra** [vɚ́ːrtəbrə] 名 椎骨

379 **multinucleated** [mʌ̀ltin(j)úːklièitid] 形 多核(性)の

380 **giant cell** [dʒáiənt sél] 名 巨細胞

> 脈瘤性骨囊胞：長骨または椎骨の内部に生じる孤立性の良性溶骨性病変．多核巨細胞を含む線維性組織に隔てられ，血液で満たされた多房性の腔から成る．

7. 囊胞性疾患

100. <u>static bone cavity</u>：An asymptomatic indentation on the lingual surface of the mandible within which a portion of the submandibular gland lies.

381 <u>static bone cavity</u> [stǽtik bóun kǽvəti]	名	静止性骨空洞
382 asymptomatic [eisìmptəmǽtik]	名	無症候性の ← symptom (582)
383 indentation [ìndèntéiʃ(ə)n]	名	陥凹
384 submandibular gland [sÀbmændíbjələr glǽnd]	名	顎下腺
385 gland [glǽnd]	名	腺

> **静止性骨空洞**：下顎骨舌側面の無症候性の陥凹で，内部に顎下腺の一部を含む．

---

101. <u>mucous cyst (=mucocele)</u>：A retention cyst resulting from obstruction of the duct of a mucous gland.

386 <u>mucous cyst</u> [mjú:kəs síst]	名	粘液囊胞
387 <u>mucocele</u> [mjú:kousì:l]	名	粘液瘤
388 mucous [mjú:kəs]	形	粘液の ← mucus (492)
389 retention cyst [riténʃ(ə)n síst]	名	貯留囊胞
390 duct [dÁkt]	名	導管
391 mucous gland [mjú:kəs glǽnd]	名	粘液腺

> **粘液囊胞(= 粘液瘤)**：粘液腺の導管の閉塞に起因する貯留囊胞．

7. 囊胞性疾患

102. ranula：A cyst in the floor of the mouth due to obstruction of the duct of the sublingual glands.

392 ranula [rǽnjələ] — 名 ガマ腫

393 sublingual gland [sÀblíŋwəl glǽnd] — 名 舌下腺

> ガマ腫：舌下腺の導管の閉塞に起因する口底の囊胞．

103. Blandin-Nuhn cyst：A cyst on the undersurface of the apex of the tongue due to obstruction of the duct of the anterior lingual glands.

394 Blandin-Nuhn cyst [blɑːndǽː núːn síst] — 名 ブランダン・ヌーン囊胞

395 apex [éipèks] — 名 尖部

396 anterior lingual gland [æntíəriər líŋwəl glǽnd] — 名 前舌腺

> ブランダン・ヌーン囊胞：前舌腺の導管の閉塞により舌尖部下面に生じる囊胞．

104. dermoid cyst：A cyst consisting of displaced ectodermal structures, the wall being formed of epithelium-lined connective tissue containing skin appendages such as sebaceous glands, sweat glands, and hair follicles.

397 dermoid cyst [də́ːrmɔid síst] — 名 類皮囊胞

398 ectodermal [èktoudə́rm(ə)l] — 形 外胚葉の

399 appendage [əpéndidʒ] — 名 付属器

400 sebaceous gland [sibéiʃəs glǽnd] — 名 脂腺

401 sweat gland [swét glǽnd] — 名 汗腺

7. 囊胞性疾患

402 □ hair follicle
[héər fálik(ə)l]

名 毛包

類皮囊胞：迷入した外胚葉組織に由来する囊胞で，壁は脂腺，汗腺，毛包等の皮膚付属器を含む結合組織から成り，上皮で裏装されている．

105. epidermoid cyst：A cyst consisting of displaced ectodermal structures, the wall being lined by keratinized stratified squamous epithelium.

403 □ epidermoid cyst
[èpədɔ́ːrmɔ̀id síst]

名 類表皮囊胞

404 □ keratinized
[kérətənàizd]

形 角化した

405 □ keratinized stratified squamous epithelium
[kérətənàizd strǽtəfàid skwéiməs èpəθíːliəm]

名 角化重層扁平上皮

類表皮囊胞：迷入した外胚葉組織に由来する囊胞で，壁は角化重層扁平上皮で裏装されている．

106. thyroglossal duct cyst (=median cervical cyst)：A cyst in the midline of the neck derived from epithelial remnants of the thyroglossal duct.

406 □ thyroglossal duct cyst
[θàiərouglás(ə)l dʌ́kt síst]

名 甲状舌管囊胞

407 □ median cervical cyst
[míːdiən sɔ́ːrvik(ə)l síst]

名 正中頸囊胞

408 □ thyroglossal duct
[θàiərouglás(ə)l dʌ́kt]

名 甲状舌管

甲状舌管囊胞(= 正中頸囊胞)：正中頸部に生じる囊胞で，甲状舌管の上皮性遺残組織に由来する．

7. 嚢胞性疾患

107. branchial cyst (=lateral cervical cyst, lymphoepithelial cyst)：A congenital cyst on the lateral part of the neck, derived from an incompletely closed branchial cleft or from parotid gland epithelium entrapped in lymph nodes during embryogenesis.

409	branchial cyst [brǽŋkiəl síst]	名 鰓嚢胞
410	lateral cervical cyst [lǽtər(ə)l sə́ːrvik(ə)l síst]	名 側頸嚢胞
411	lymphoepithelial cyst [lìmfouèpəθíːliəl síst]	名 リンパ上皮性嚢胞
412	branchial cleft [brǽŋkiəl kléft]	名 鰓裂
413	parotid gland [pərátəd glǽnd]	名 耳下腺
414	embryogenesis [èmbrioudʒénəsəs]	名 胚発生

鰓嚢胞(= 側頸嚢胞，リンパ上皮性嚢胞)：側頸部に生じる先天性の嚢胞で，胚発生期の鰓裂の閉鎖不全または耳下腺上皮のリンパ節内迷入に由来する．

---

108. postoperative maxillary cyst：A cyst that occurs as a delayed complication of radical surgery of the maxillary sinus 10 to 20 years later.

415	postoperative maxillary cyst [pòustápərətiv mǽksəlèri síst]	名 術後性上顎嚢胞
416	complication [kàmpləkéiʃ(ə)n]	名 合併症
417	radical surgery [rǽdik(ə)l sə́ːrdʒəri]	名 根治手術
418	surgery [sə́ːrdʒəri]	名 手術，外科的処置

術後性上顎嚢胞：上顎洞の根治手術の遅発合併症として 10 から 20 年後に生じる嚢胞．

8 腫瘍および腫瘍類似疾患

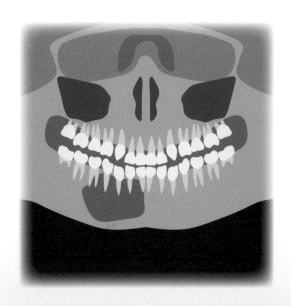

8. 腫瘍および腫瘍類似疾患

109. ameloblastoma: A benign odontogenic tumor of epithelial origin that occurs most commonly in the molar-ramus region of the mandible.

419 □ ameloblastoma
[æ̀məloublǽstóumə]

名 エナメル上皮腫

420 □ ramus
[réiməs]

名 下顎枝

エナメル上皮腫：上皮由来の良性の歯原性腫瘍で，下顎大臼歯部から下顎枝部にかけて好発する．

110. keratocystic odontogenic tumor: A benign cystic tumor lined with parakeratinized stratified squamous epithelium that most often affects the molar-ramus region of the mandible.

421 □ keratocystic odontogenic tumor
[kèrətousístik oudàntoudʒénik t(j)úːmər]

名 角化嚢胞性歯原性腫瘍

422 □ parakeratinized
[pæ̀rəkérətənàizd]

形 錯角化の ← keratinized (404)

角化嚢胞性歯原性腫瘍：錯角化重層扁平上皮で裏装された良性の嚢胞性腫瘍で，下顎大臼歯部から下顎枝部にかけて好発する．

111. adenomatoid odontogenic tumor: A benign epithelial tumor that affects young individuals with a female predominance, appearing radiographically as a well-circumscribed unilocular radiolucency usually surrounding the crown of an impacted tooth.

423 □ adenomatoid odontogenic tumor
[æ̀dənóumətɔ̀id oudàntoudʒénik t(j)úːmər]

名 腺腫様歯原性腫瘍

424 □ well-circumscribed
[wél sə́ːrkəmskràibd]

形 境界明瞭な

425 □ radiolucency
[rèidioulúːsənsi]

名 エックス線透過像 ← radiolucent (461)

腺腫様歯原性腫瘍：若者，とくに女性に好発する良性の上皮性腫瘍で，エックス線写真では，通常，埋伏歯の歯冠を取り囲む境界明瞭な単房性透過像を呈する．

8. 腫瘍および腫瘍類似疾患

112. <u>calcifying epithelial odontogenic tumor</u>: A benign intraosseous tumor of epithelial origin characterized by proliferation of polygonal epithelial cells and calcified amyloid-like deposits.

426 <u>calcifying epithelial odontogenic tumor</u> [kǽlsəfàiiŋ èpəθí:liəl oudàntoudʒénik t(j)ú:mər]	名 石灰化上皮性歯原性腫瘍
427 intraosseous [ìntrəásiəs]	形 骨内(性)の
428 proliferation [prəlìfəréiʃ(ə)n]	名 増殖
429 amyloid [ǽməlɔ̀id]	名 アミロイド
430 deposit [dipázət]	名 沈着物

<u>石灰化上皮性歯原性腫瘍</u>：上皮由来の良性の骨内性腫瘍で，多角形の上皮性細胞の増殖と石灰化したアミロイド様沈着物を特徴とする．

---

113. <u>ameloblastic fibroma</u>: A benign odontogenic tumor characterized by proliferation of both epithelial and mesenchymal components of the tooth bud without the production of dental hard tissue, occurring most commonly in the mandibles of children and adolescents.

431 <u>ameloblastic fibroma</u> [æ̀məloublǽstik faibróumə]	名 エナメル上皮線維腫
432 ameloblastic [æ̀məloublǽstik]	形 エナメル芽細胞の ← ameloblast (994)
433 fibroma [faibróumə]	名 線維腫
434 mesenchymal [məzéŋkəməl]	形 間葉性の
435 tooth bud [tú:θ bʌ́d]	名 歯蕾
436 hard tissue [há:rd tíʃu]	名 硬組織

<u>エナメル上皮線維腫</u>：歯蕾の上皮成分および間葉成分の増殖を特徴とする良性の歯原性腫瘍で，歯牙硬組織形成をともなわない．青少年の下顎に好発する．

8. 腫瘍および腫瘍類似疾患

114. odontoma: A hamartomatous odontogenic tumor consisting of cementum, dentin, and enamel that may be arranged in the form of teeth (compound odontoma) or as an unrecognizable mass (complex odontoma).

437 **odontoma** [òudɑntóumə] — 名 歯牙腫

438 **hamartomatous** [hæmɑ̀ːrtóumətəs] — 形 過誤腫性の ← hamartoma (995)

439 **compound odontoma** [kámpàund òudɑntóumə] — 名 集合性歯牙腫

440 **complex odontoma** [kámplèks òudɑntóumə] — 名 複雑性歯牙腫

> 歯牙腫：過誤腫性の歯原性腫瘍で，セメント質，象牙質，エナメル質が歯の形に配列しているもの（集合性歯牙種）と，識別不能な塊となっているもの（複雑性歯牙種）とがある．

115. calcifying cystic odontogenic tumor: A benign intraosseous tumor of the jaw with a cystic architecture, characterized by the presence of ghost cells within the lesion.

441 **calcifying cystic odontogenic tumor** [kǽlsəfàiiŋ sístik oudàntoudʒénik t(j)úːmər] — 名 石灰化囊胞性歯原性腫瘍

442 **ghost cell** [góust sél] — 名 幻影細胞

> 石灰化囊胞性歯原性腫瘍：顎骨内に生じる良性腫瘍で，囊胞状の形態を示す．病変内部の幻影細胞を特徴とする．

116. odontogenic fibroma: A benign fibroblastic tumor arising from the dental papilla, the dental follicle, or the periodontal membrane, most commonly found in the mandibular molar area, and composed of fibrous connective tissue and odontogenic epithelium.

443 **odontogenic fibroma** [oudàntoudʒénik faibróumə] — 名 歯原性線維腫

444 **fibroblastic** [fàibroublǽstik] — 形 線維芽細胞（性）の

8. 腫瘍および腫瘍類似疾患

445 ☐ **dental papilla**
[dént(ə)l pəpílə]

名 歯乳頭

446 ☐ **dental follicle**
[dént(ə)l fálik(ə)l]

名 歯小嚢

447 ☐ **fibrous connective tissue**
[fáibrəs kənéktiv tíʃu]

名 線維性結合組織

> **歯原性線維腫**：歯乳頭，歯小嚢，または歯根膜由来の良性の線維芽細胞性腫瘍．下顎大臼歯部に好発し，線維性結合組織および歯原性上皮から成る．

---

117. <u>odontogenic myxoma</u>：A benign but locally invasive intraosseous tumor of the jaw consisting of loosely arranged spindle, stellate-shaped, or round cells in a myxoid stroma.

448 ☐ <u>**odontogenic myxoma**</u>
[oudàntoudʒénik miksóumə]

名 歯原性粘液腫

449 ☐ **myxoma**
[miksóumə]

名 粘液腫

450 ☐ **invasive**
[invéisiv]

形 浸潤性の

451 ☐ **myxoid**
[míksɔ̀id]

形 粘液様の

452 ☐ **stroma**
[stróumə]

名 基質

> **歯原性粘液腫**：顎骨内に生じる局所浸潤性の良性腫瘍．粘液様基質の中に紡錘形・星形・円形の細胞がまばらに配列している．

---

118. <u>cementoblastoma</u>：A benign tumor of the cementum that primarily affects the mandibular molar area, characterized by proliferation of cementum-like tissue that is attached to the roots of teeth.

453 ☐ <u>**cementoblastoma**</u>
[simèntoublæstóumə]

名 セメント芽細胞腫

> **セメント芽細胞腫**：下顎大臼歯部に好発するセメント質の良性腫瘍で，増殖したセメント質様組織の歯根への癒着を特徴とする．

8. 腫瘍および腫瘍類似疾患

119. primary intraosseous squamous cell carcinoma：An odontogenic malignant tumor that develops from residual odontogenic epithelium, a keratocystic odontogenic tumor, or an odontogenic cyst.

454 primary intraosseous squamous cell carcinoma
[práimèri ìntrəásiəs skwéiməs sél kà:rsənóumə]
名 原発性骨内扁平上皮癌

455 primary
[práimèri]
形 原発性の

456 squamous cell
[skwéiməs sél]
名 扁平上皮細胞

457 carcinoma
[kà:rsənóumə]
名 癌

458 malignant
[məlígnənt]
形 悪性の ↔ benign (370)

原発性骨内扁平上皮癌：遺残した歯原性上皮，角化嚢胞性歯原性腫瘍，または歯原性嚢胞に由来する歯原性悪性腫瘍．

120. ameloblastic fibrosarcoma：A rapidly growing, painful, radiolucent odontogenic tumor that usually arises through malignant change in the mesenchymal tissue of a preexisting ameloblastic fibroma.

459 ameloblastic fibrosarcoma
[æməloublǽstik fàibrousɑ:rkóumə]
名 エナメル上皮線維肉腫

460 fibrosarcoma
[fàibrousɑ:rkóumə]
名 線維肉腫

461 radiolucent
[rèidioulú:sənt]
形 エックス線透過性の

エナメル上皮線維肉腫：急速に増殖する歯原性腫瘍で，疼痛をともない，エックス線透過性である．通常，既存のエナメル上皮線維腫の間葉性組織の悪性転化に由来する．

121. pleomorphic adenoma：A benign tumor composed of the epithelial and mesenchymal elements of the salivary gland.

8. 腫瘍および腫瘍類似疾患

462 □ **pleomorphic adenoma**
[plì:oumɔ́:rfik ædənóumə]

名 多形腺腫

463 □ **adenoma**
[ædənóumə]

名 腺腫

464 □ **salivary gland**
[sǽləvèri glǽnd]

名 唾液腺

多形腺腫：唾液腺の上皮成分と間葉成分から構成される良性腫瘍．

---

122. Warthin tumor：A benign tumor of the parotid gland composed of a papillary proliferation of epithelial cells with lymphoid tissue.

465 □ **Warthin tumor**
[wɔ́:rθən t(j)ú:mər]

名 ウォーシン腫瘍

466 □ **papillary**
[pǽpəlèri]

形 乳頭(状)の ← papilla (185)

467 □ **lymphoid tissue**
[límfɔid tíʃu]

名 リンパ組織

ウォーシン腫瘍：上皮細胞の乳頭状増殖とリンパ組織から構成される耳下腺の良性腫瘍．

---

123. oncocytoma：A benign tumor that primarily affects the parotid gland, composed of large cells with cytoplasm that is granular and eosinophilic because of the presence of abundant mitochondria.

468 □ **oncocytoma**
[ùnkousaitóumə]

名 オンコサイトーマ

469 □ **cytoplasm**
[sáitouplæ̀zm]

名 細胞質

470 □ **granular**
[grǽnjələr]

形 顆粒状の

471 □ **eosinophilic**
[ì:əsìnəfílik]

形 好酸性の

472 □ **mitochondria**
[màitəkándriə]

名 ミトコンドリア（複; 単 mitochondrion [màitəkándriən]）

オンコサイトーマ：耳下腺に好発する良性腫瘍．大型の細胞から成り，その細胞質は多くのミトコンドリアを含むため顆粒状で好酸性となる．

8. 腫瘍および腫瘍類似疾患

124. benign lymphoepithelial lesion: A chronic disorder of unknown etiology that affects the lacrimal and salivary glands, characterized by lymphocyte infiltration, the formation of epimyoepithelial islands, and atrophy of the gland parenchyma.

473	benign lymphoepithelial lesion [bináin lìmfouèpəθí:liəl lí:ʒ(ə)n]	名 良性リンパ上皮性病変
474	etiology [ì:tiálədʒi]	名 原因,病因
475	lacrimal gland [lǽkrəm(ə)l glǽnd]	名 涙腺
476	lymphocyte [límfousàit]	名 リンパ球
477	infiltration [ìnfiltréiʃ(ə)n]	名 浸潤
478	epimyoepithelial island [èpəmàiouèpəθí:liəl áilənd]	名 筋上皮島
479	parenchyma [pəréŋkəmə]	名 実質

良性リンパ上皮性病変:涙腺や唾液腺に生じる原因不明の慢性疾患.リンパ球浸潤,筋上皮島形成,腺実質の萎縮等を特徴とする.

---

125. chronic sclerosing submandibular sialadenitis (=Küttner's tumor): A chronic inflammation of the submandibular gland characterized by periductal sclerosis, acinar atrophy, and lymphocyte infiltration.

480	chronic sclerosing submandibular sialadenitis [kránik skləróusiŋ sʌ̀bmændíbjələr sàiəlǽdənáitəs]	名 慢性硬化性顎下腺炎
481	Küttner's tumor [k(j)ú:tnərz t(j)ú:mər]	名 キュットナー腫瘍
482	sialadenitis [sàiəlǽdənáitəs]	名 唾液腺炎
483	periductal [pèridʌ́kt(ə)l]	形 導管周囲の

8. 腫瘍および腫瘍類似疾患

484 □ sclerosis
[skləróusəs]

名 硬化

485 □ acinar
[ǽsənər]

形 腺房の

慢性硬化性顎下腺炎(= キュットナー腫瘍)：顎下腺の慢性の炎症で，導管周囲の硬化，腺房の萎縮，リンパ球浸潤等を特徴とする．

---

126. oral cancer：Any malignant neoplasm located in the oral cavity, which most commonly involves the tongue but may also occur on the floor of the mouth, buccal mucosa, gingiva, lips, or palate.

486 □ oral cancer
[ɔ́:r(ə)l kǽnsər]

名 口腔癌

487 □ cancer
[kǽnsər]

名 癌

488 □ neoplasm
[ní:ouplæzm]

名 新生物

489 □ buccal mucosa
[bʌ́k(ə)l mjukóusə]

名 頬粘膜

口腔癌：口腔内に生じる悪性新生物の総称．発生部位は舌がもっとも多く，他に口底，頬粘膜，歯肉，口唇，口蓋にも見られる．

---

127. adenoid cystic carcinoma：A histologic type of carcinoma characterized by large epithelial masses containing round, glandlike spaces that contain mucus, occurring in the salivary and mammary glands, and mucous glands of the respiratory tract.

490 □ adenoid cystic carcinoma
[ǽdənɔ̀id sístik kà:rsənóumə]

名 腺様嚢胞癌

491 □ histologic
[hìstəládʒik]

形 組織学の

492 □ mucus
[mjú:kəs]

名 粘液

493 □ mammary gland
[mǽməri glǽnd]

名 乳腺

494 □ respiratory tract
[réspərətɔ̀:ri trǽkt]

名 気道

8. 腫瘍および腫瘍類似疾患

> **腺様嚢胞癌**：粘液を含む丸い腺様の腔を有する大型の上皮塊を特徴とする癌の一組織型．唾液腺，乳腺，気道の粘液腺等に生じる．

128. **mucoepidermoid carcinoma**: A malignant tumor of glandular tissues, especially the ducts of the salivary glands, composed of mucous, epidermoid, and intermediate cells.

495 □ **mucoepidermoid carcinoma**
[mjùːkouèpədɔ́ːrmɔ̀id kɑ̀ːrsənóumə]
【名】粘表皮癌

496 □ **glandular tissue**
[glǽndʒələr tíʃu]
【名】腺組織

497 □ **mucous cell**
[mjúːkəs sél]
【名】粘液細胞

498 □ **epidermoid cell**
[èpədɔ́ːrmɔ̀id sél]
【名】類表皮細胞

499 □ **intermediate cell**
[ìntərmíːdièit sél]
【名】中間細胞

> **粘表皮癌**：腺組織，とくに唾液腺の導管に生じる悪性腫瘍．粘液細胞，類表皮細胞，中間細胞から構成される．

129. **acinic cell carcinoma**: A low-grade, slowly growing salivary gland carcinoma with serous acinar cell differentiation.

500 □ **acinic cell carcinoma**
[əsínik sél kɑ̀ːrsənóumə]
【名】腺房細胞癌

501 □ **low-grade**
[lóu gréid]
【形】低悪性度の

502 □ **serous**
[síərəs]
【形】漿液(性)の ← serum (961)

503 □ **acinar cell**
[ǽsənər sél]
【名】腺房細胞

504 □ **differentiation**
[dìfərènʃiéiʃ(ə)n]
【名】分化

> **腺房細胞癌**：悪性度が低く進行の遅い唾液腺の癌で，漿液性腺房細胞への分化を示す．

8. 腫瘍および腫瘍類似疾患

> **130. epulis**: A nonspecific term used for a localized gingival growth. The classification includes epulis granulomatosa, fibromatous epulis, ossifying epulis, giant cell epulis, pregnancy epulis, and congenital epulis.

505 epulis [ipjú:ləs] — 名 エプーリス

506 growth [gróuθ] — 名 増殖(物)

507 epulis granulomatosa [ipjú:ləs grænjəlòumətóusə] — 名 肉芽腫性エプーリス

508 fibromatous epulis [faibrámətəs ipjú:ləs] — 名 線維腫性エプーリス

509 ossifying epulis [ásəfàiiŋ ipjú:ləs] — 名 骨形成性エプーリス

510 giant cell epulis [dʒáiənt sél ipjú:ləs] — 名 巨細胞性エプーリス

511 pregnancy epulis [prégnənsi ipjú:ləs] — 名 妊娠性エプーリス

512 congenital epulis [kəndʒénit(ə)l ipjú:ləs] — 名 先天性エプーリス

> **エプーリス**：歯肉に生じる限局性増殖物の慣用名．肉芽腫性エプーリス，線維腫性エプーリス，骨形成性エプーリス，巨細胞性エプーリス，妊娠性エプーリス，先天性エプーリス等に分類される．

> **131. denture fibroma**: Hyperplasia of fibrous connective tissue due to chronic mechanical irritation by the flange of a poorly fitting denture.

513 denture fibroma [déntʃər faibróumə] — 名 義歯性線維腫

514 denture [déntʃər] — 名 義歯

515 flange [flǽndʒ] — 名 フレンジ，義歯床翼部

> **義歯性線維腫**：不適合な義歯のフレンジによる慢性的な物理的刺激に起因する線維性結合組織の増殖．

8. 腫瘍および腫瘍類似疾患

132. palatal torus: A benign bony growth occurring in the midline of the hard palate.

516 □ palatal torus
[pǽlət(ə)l tɔ́:rəs]
名 口蓋隆起

517 □ torus
[tɔ́:rəs]
名 隆起

口蓋隆起：硬口蓋の正中部に生じる良性の骨質増殖物．

133. mandibular torus: A benign bony growth appearing on the lingual aspect of the mandibular premolar region.

518 □ mandibular torus
[mændíbjələr tɔ́:rəs]
名 下顎隆起

下顎隆起：下顎小臼歯部の舌側に生じる良性の骨質増殖物．

134. osseous dysplasia: A benign fibro-osseous lesion of the jaw composed of fibrous connective tissue containing cementum-like material.

519 □ osseous dysplasia
[ásiəs displéiʒ(i)ə]
名 骨性異形成症

520 □ dysplasia
[displéiʒ(i)ə]
名 異形成(症)

521 □ fibro-osseous
[fáibrou ásiəs]
形 線維骨性の

骨性異形成症：顎骨に生じる良性の線維骨性病変で，セメント質様物質を含む線維性結合組織から成る．

135. McCune-Albright syndrome: Polyostotic fibrous dysplasia with brown patches of pigmentation and endocrine dysfunction, especially precocious puberty in girls.

522 □ McCune-Albright syndrome
[mək(j)ú:n ɔ́:lbràit síndròum]
名 マッキューン・オールブライト症候群

523 □ syndrome
[síndròum]
名 症候群

8. 腫瘍および腫瘍類似疾患

⁵²⁴☐ polyostotic fibrous dysplasia
[pàliɑstɑ́tik fáibrəs displéiʒ(i)ə]

名 多骨性線維性異形成症

⁵²⁵☐ pigmentation
[pìgməntéiʃ(ə)n]

名 色素沈着

⁵²⁶☐ dysfunction
[disfʌ́ŋkʃ(ə)n]

名 機能障害，機能不全

⁵²⁷☐ precocious puberty
[prikóuʃəs pjúːbərti]

名 思春期早発症

⁵²⁸☐ puberty
[pjúːbərti]

名 思春期

> **マッキューン・オールブライト症候群**：褐色の色素沈着斑と内分泌機能障害，とくに女児における思春期早発症をともなう多骨性線維性異形成症．

136. cherubism: Progressive, symmetric, and painless swelling of the jaw beginning in early childhood due to hereditary giant cell lesions, manifested radiographically as multilocular radiolucencies.

⁵²⁹☐ cherubism
[tʃérəbìzm]

名 ケルビズム

> **ケルビズム**：小児期早期に初発する顎骨の進行性，対称性，無痛性の腫脹．遺伝性の巨細胞性病変に起因し，エックス線写真では多房性透過像を呈する．

137. Langerhans cell histiocytosis: Proliferation of Langerhans cells with infiltration into organs, clinically divided into three groups: unifocal, multifocal unisystem, and multifocal multisystem.

⁵³⁰☐ Langerhans cell histiocytosis
[láːŋərhàːns sél hìstiousaitóusəs]

名 ランゲルハンス細胞組織球症

⁵³¹☐ unifocal
[jùːnifóuk(ə)l]

形 単病巣性の

⁵³²☐ multifocal
[mʌ̀ltifóuk(ə)l]

形 多病巣性の

> **ランゲルハンス細胞組織球症**：臓器浸潤をともなうランゲルハンス細胞の増殖で，臨床的に単病巣性，多病巣性・単一臓器性，多病巣性・多臓器性の3グループに分類される．

9 口腔粘膜疾患

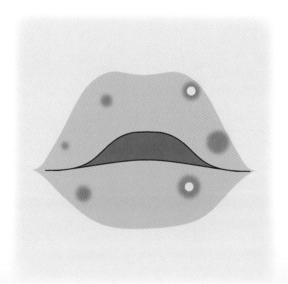

9. 口腔粘膜疾患

138. herpetic gingivostomatitis: Vesicular lesions of the gingiva and oral mucosa that progress to erosions and ulcers, caused by primary infection of herpes simplex virus type one.

533 herpetic gingivostomatitis [hərpétik dʒìndʒəvoustòumətáitəs] — 名 ヘルペス性歯肉口内炎,疱疹性歯肉口内炎

534 herpetic [hərpétik] — 形 ヘルペス(性)の ← herpes (539)

535 gingivostomatitis [dʒìndʒəvoustòumətáitəs] — 名 歯肉口内炎

536 vesicular [vəsíkjələr] — 形 小水疱(性)の ← vesicle (543)

537 erosion [iróuʒ(ə)n] — 名 びらん

538 ulcer [́́lsər] — 名 潰瘍

539 herpes [hə́ːrpiz] — 名 ヘルペス

540 herpes simplex virus [hə́ːrpiz símplèks váiərəs] — 名 単純ヘルペスウイルス

541 virus [váiərəs] — 名 ウイルス

> **ヘルペス性歯肉口内炎(＝疱疹性歯肉口内炎)**：歯肉および口腔粘膜の小水疱性病変で，びらん，潰瘍へと進行する．単純ヘルペスウイルス1型の初感染に起因する．

139. herpes labialis: An infection by herpes simplex virus type one, resulting in clusters of vesicles on the lips and the perioral skin.

542 herpes labialis [hə́ːrpiz lèibiǽləs] — 名 口唇ヘルペス

543 vesicle [vésik(ə)l] — 名 小水疱

544 perioral [pèrióːr(ə)l] — 形 口周囲の

> **口唇ヘルペス**：単純ヘルペスウイルス1型による感染症で，口唇および口周囲の皮膚に集簇性の小水疱を形成する．

9. 口腔粘膜疾患

140. herpes zoster: An acute disease caused by reactivation of the latent varicella-zoster virus, characterized by neuralgic pain and vesicular eruptions in the areas supplied by the sensory nerves.

#	英語	品詞	日本語
545	herpes zoster [hə́ːrpiz zástər]	名	帯状疱疹
546	reactivation [riæktəvéiʃ(ə)n]	名	再活性化
547	latent [léitənt]	形	潜伏(性)の
548	varicella-zoster virus [værəsélə zástər váiərəs]	名	水痘・帯状疱疹ウイルス
549	neuralgic [n(j)uərǽldʒik]	形	神経痛の ← neuralgia (791)
550	eruption [irʌ́pʃ(ə)n]	名	発疹
551	sensory nerve [sénsəri nə́ːrv]	名	感覚神経
552	nerve [nə́ːrv]	名	神経

帯状疱疹：潜伏感染していた水痘・帯状疱疹ウイルスの再活性化に起因する急性疾患．感覚神経の分布領域における神経痛様疼痛と小水疱性発疹を特徴とする．

141. herpangina: An infection caused mainly by coxsackievirus A, resulting in vesicular lesions on the soft palate and fauces, sore throat, dysphagia, and fever.

#	英語	品詞	日本語
553	herpangina [hə̀ːrpændʒáinə]	名	ヘルパンギーナ
554	coxsackievirus [kɑksǽkivàiərəs]	名	コクサッキーウイルス
555	fauces [fɔ́ːsìːz]	名	口峡
556	sore throat [sɔ́ːr θróut]	名	咽頭痛

9. 口腔粘膜疾患

557 **dysphagia**
[disféidʒ(i)ə]

名 嚥下困難

> ヘルパンギーナ：コクサッキーウイルスA群を主な原因とする感染症で，軟口蓋および口峡の小水疱性病変，咽頭痛，嚥下困難，発熱等をともなう．

142. hand-foot-and-mouth disease： An infection caused mainly by coxsackievirus A16 and enterovirus 71, resulting in vesicular lesions in the mouth, on the hands and feet.

558 **hand-foot-and-mouth disease**
[hǽnd fút ənd máuθ dizíːz]

名 手足口病

559 **enterovirus**
[èntərouváiərəs]

名 エンテロウイルス

> 手足口病：コクサッキーウイルスA16およびエンテロウイルス71を主な原因とする感染症で，口腔，手，足に小水疱性病変を形成する．

143. Koplik spots： Small white spots, each surrounded by a red ring, that occur on the buccal mucosa in the early phase of measles.

560 **Koplik spots**
[káplik spáts]

名 コプリック斑

561 **measles**
[míːz(ə)lz]

名 麻疹

> コプリック斑：麻疹の初期に頬粘膜に生じる小白斑で，周囲に紅暈をともなう．

144. pemphigus： An autoimmune disease in which autoantibodies are produced against intercellular adhesion molecules, causing bullae and erosions on the skin and mucous membrane.

562 **pemphigus**
[pémfigəs]

名 天疱瘡

563 **autoimmune**
[ɔ̀ːtouimjúːn]

形 自己免疫の

564 **autoimmune disease**
[ɔ̀ːtouimjúːn dizíːz]

名 自己免疫疾患

9. 口腔粘膜疾患

565 **autoantibody**
[ɔ̀:touǽntibɑ̀di]
名 自己抗体 ← antibody (996)

566 **intercellular adhesion molecule**
[ìntərséljələr ædhí:ʒ(ə)n málikjù:l]
名 細胞間接着分子

567 **molecule**
[málikjù:l]
名 分子

568 **bullae**
[búlì:]
名 水疱（複）；単 bulla[búlə]）

569 **mucous membrane**
[mjú:kəs mémbrèin]
名 粘膜 = mucosa (194)

> **天疱瘡**：細胞間接着分子に対する自己抗体が産生され，皮膚や粘膜に水疱とびらんを生じる自己免疫疾患．

145. pemphigoid：An autoimmune mucocutaneous disease of elderly persons characterized by chronic, pruritic bullae.

570 **pemphigoid**
[pémfəgɔ̀id]
名 類天疱瘡

571 **mucocutaneous**
[mjù:koukjutéiniəs]
形 粘膜と皮膚の

572 **pruritic**
[prurítik]
形 掻痒性の

> **類天疱瘡**：高齢者に好発する自己免疫性皮膚粘膜疾患で，慢性の掻痒性水疱を特徴とする．

146. epidermolysis bullosa：A group of hereditary chronic mucocutaneous diseases in which bullae and erosions result from slight mechanical trauma.

573 **epidermolysis bullosa**
[èpədərmáləsəs bulóusə]
名 表皮水疱症

> **表皮水疱症**：軽微な物理的外傷によって水疱やびらんを生じる遺伝性の慢性皮膚粘膜疾患の一群．

9. 口腔粘膜疾患

147. erythema multiforme：An acute inflammatory mucocutaneous disease characterized by red edematous papules and bullae.

574 erythema multiforme [èrəθíːmə mÀltəfɔ́ːrmi]	名 多形紅斑
575 edematous [idémətəs]	形 浮腫(性)の ← edema (249)
576 papule [pæpjul]	名 丘疹

多形紅斑：赤い浮腫性丘疹と水疱を特徴とする急性の炎症性皮膚粘膜疾患.

148. Stevens-Johnson syndrome：A severe form of erythema multiforme in which the lesions may involve the mucous membranes of the mouth, nostrils, eyes, anus, and genitals, accompanied by such systemic symptoms as malaise, headache, fever, and arthralgia.

577 Stevens-Johnson syndrome [stíːv(ə)nz dʒáns(ə)n síndròum]	名 スティーヴンズ・ジョンソン症候群
578 nostril [nástr(ə)l]	名 鼻孔
579 anus [éinəs]	名 肛門
580 genitals [dʒénət(ə)lz]	名 生殖器（複；通常は複数形を使用する）
581 systemic [sistémik]	形 全身(性)の
582 symptom [símptəm]	名 症状
583 malaise [məléiz]	名 倦怠感
584 headache [hédèik]	名 頭痛
585 arthralgia [ɑːrθrǽldʒ(i)ə]	名 関節痛

スティーヴンズ・ジョンソン症候群：多形紅斑の重症型. 病変は口腔, 鼻孔, 目, 肛門, 生殖器の粘膜に及び, 倦怠感, 頭痛, 発熱, 関節痛等の全身症状をともなう.

9. 口腔粘膜疾患

149. toxic epidermal necrolysis (TEN)：A severe drug hypersensitivity characterized by widespread epidermal erythema, necrosis, and bullous detachment.

586 **toxic epidermal necrolysis (TEN)**
[táksik èpədə́ːrm(ə)l nekráləsəs]
名 中毒性表皮壊死症

587 **epidermal**
[èpədə́ːrm(ə)l]
形 表皮の ← epidermis (997)

588 **bullous**
[búləs]
形 水疱(性)の ← bulla (568)

589 **detachment**
[ditǽtʃmənt]
名 剥離

中毒性表皮壊死症：広範囲に及ぶ表皮の紅斑，壊死，水疱性剥離を特徴とする重篤な薬物過敏症．

150. systemic lupus erythematosus (SLE)：A systemic autoimmune disease with variable features, frequently including fever, arthritis, erythema, pleuritis, pericarditis, renal lesions, and anemia.

590 **systemic lupus erythematosus (SLE)**
[sistémik lúːpəs èrəθìːmətóusəs]
名 全身性エリテマトーデス

591 **arthritis**
[ɑːrθráitəs]
名 関節炎

592 **pleuritis**
[pluəráitəs]
名 胸膜炎

593 **pericarditis**
[pèrikɑːrdáitəs]
名 心膜炎

594 **renal**
[ríːn(ə)l]
形 腎臓の

595 **anemia**
[əníːmiə]
名 貧血

全身性エリテマトーデス：多彩な症状を示す全身性の自己免疫疾患．しばしば発熱，関節炎，紅斑，胸膜炎，心膜炎，腎病変，貧血等をともなう．

9. 口腔粘膜疾患

151. <u>discoid lupus erythematosus (DLE)</u>: A superficial inflammation of the skin that appears on light-exposed areas such as the face, scalp, and ears, characterized by red discoid macules that progress to atrophic scars.

596 <u>discoid lupus erythematosus (DLE)</u> [dískɔ̀id lúːpəs èrəθìːmətóusəs]	名 円板状エリテマトーデス
597 scalp [skǽlp]	名 頭皮
598 macule [mǽkjul]	名 斑
599 atrophic [ətráfik]	形 萎縮(性)の ← atrophy (176)
600 scar [skáːr]	名 瘢痕

<u>円板状エリテマトーデス</u>：顔面，頭皮，耳等の露光部位に生じる皮膚表面の炎症．赤い円板状の斑を特徴とし，萎縮性瘢痕へと進行する．

---

152. <u>angioedema (=Quincke's edema)</u>: Localized edema caused by dilatation and increased permeability of the capillaries, characterized by the development of giant wheals.

601 <u>angioedema</u> [æ̀ndʒiouidíːmə]	名 血管性浮腫
602 <u>Quincke's edema</u> [kvíŋkəz idíːmə]	名 クインケ浮腫
603 dilatation [dìlətéiʃ(ə)n]	名 拡張
604 permeability [pə̀ːrmiəbíləti]	名 透過性
605 capillary [kǽpəlèri]	名 毛細血管
606 wheal [(h)wíːl]	名 膨疹

<u>血管性浮腫(＝クインケ浮腫)</u>：毛細血管の拡張と透過性亢進に起因する限局性の浮腫．巨大な膨疹の発生を特徴とする．

9. 口腔粘膜疾患

153. recurrent aphthous stomatitis：A recurrent disease of unknown etiology, characterized by small round ulcers on the oral mucosa covered by a grayish exudate.

607 recurrent aphthous stomatitis
[rikə́:rənt ǽfθəs stòumətáitəs]
名 再発性アフタ性口内炎

608 recurrent
[rikə́:rənt]
形 再発(性)の

609 aphthous
[ǽfθəs]
形 アフタ(性)の ← aphtha (698)

610 exudate
[éks(j)udèit]
名 滲出物

> 再発性アフタ性口内炎：原因不明の再発性疾患．灰色の滲出物に覆われた口腔粘膜上の円形の小潰瘍を特徴とする．

154. Behçet disease：A chronic disorder with prominent mucosal inflammation characterized by recurrent oral and genital ulcers, uveitis, and erythema nodosum.

611 Behçet disease
[béitʃet dizí:z]
名 ベーチェット病

612 genital
[dʒénət(ə)l]
形 生殖器の，陰部の

613 uveitis
[jù:viáitəs]
名 ブドウ膜炎

614 erythema nodosum
[èrəθí:mə noudóusəm]
名 結節性紅斑

> ベーチェット病：顕著な粘膜炎症をともなう慢性疾患．再発性の口腔・陰部潰瘍，ブドウ膜炎，結節性紅斑等を特徴とする．

9. 口腔粘膜疾患

155. gangrenous stomatitis (=noma): A gangrenous inflammation, usually beginning in the mucous membrane of the angle of the mouth or cheek, and then progressing fairly rapidly to involve the entire lips or cheek, with conspicuous necrosis and sloughing of tissue.

615 □ **gangrenous stomatitis**
[gǽŋgrənəs stòumətáitəs]
名 壊疽性口内炎

616 □ **noma**
[nóumə]
名 水癌

617 □ **gangrenous**
[gǽŋgrənəs]
形 壊疽(性)の ← gangrene (998)

618 □ **angle of mouth**
[ǽŋgl əv máuθ]
名 口角

> 壊疽性口内炎(＝水癌)：通常，口角または頬の粘膜から始まり，口唇または頬全体に急速に広がる壊疽性の炎症．組織の壊死や脱落が顕著に見られる．

---

156. stomatitis medicamentosa: Inflammation of the oral mucosa associated with a systemic drug allergy; lesions may consist of erythema, vesicles, bullae, ulcers, or angioedema.

619 □ **stomatitis medicamentosa**
[stòumətáitəs mədìkəmentóusə]
名 薬物性口内炎

620 □ **allergy**
[ǽlərdʒi]
名 アレルギー

> 薬物性口内炎：全身性の薬物アレルギーに関連する口腔粘膜の炎症．紅斑，小水疱，水疱，潰瘍，血管性浮腫等の病変を呈する．

---

157. oral lichen planus: A recurrent, pruritic, inflammatory eruption that affects the oral mucosa, clinically classified as reticular, papular, plaque-like, erosive, atrophic, and bullous types.

621 □ **oral lichen planus**
[ɔ́:r(ə)l láikən pléinəs]
名 口腔扁平苔癬

622 □ **lichen**
[láikən]
名 苔癬

623 □ **lichen planus**
[láikən pléinəs]
名 扁平苔癬

9. 口腔粘膜疾患

624 □ **reticular**
[ritíkjələr]
形 網状の

625 □ **papular**
[pǽpjələr]
形 丘疹(性)の ← papule (576)

626 □ **plaque**
[plǽk]
名 斑

627 □ **erosive**
[iróusiv]
形 びらん(性)の ← erosion (537)

> 口腔扁平苔癬：口腔粘膜に生じる再発性，搔痒性，炎症性の発疹．臨床的に，網状型，丘疹型，白斑型，びらん型，萎縮型，水疱型に分類される．

158. oral candidiasis：An infection caused by *Candida albicans* characterized by white or red plaques on inner cheeks, tongue, or lips.

628 □ **oral candidiasis**
[ɔ́ːr(ə)l kændədáiəsəs]
名 口腔カンジダ症

629 □ **candidiasis**
[kændədáiəsəs]
名 カンジダ症

630 □ *Candida albicans*
[kǽndədə ǽlbəkænz]
名 カンジダ・アルビカンス

> 口腔カンジダ症：頬の内側，舌，口唇等に生じる白斑または紅斑を特徴とするカンジダ・アルビカンスによる感染症．

159. leukoplakia：A precancerous white plaque on the oral mucosa caused by hyperkeratosis.

631 □ **leukoplakia**
[lùːkoupléikiə]
名 白板症

632 □ **precancerous**
[priːkǽnsərəs]
形 前癌性の ← cancer (487)

633 □ **hyperkeratosis**
[hàipərkèrətóusəs]
名 角質増殖 ← keratosis (968)

> 白板症：角質増殖に起因する口腔粘膜上の前癌性白斑．

9. 口腔粘膜疾患

160. erythroplakia : A precancerous red plaque on the oral mucosa with a velvet appearance.

634 ☐ erythroplakia
[irìθroupléikiə]

名 紅板症

紅板症：ビロード状の外観をもつ口腔粘膜上の前癌性紅斑.

---

161. hairy leukoplakia : A white lesion with a hairy surface appearing on the tongue and buccal mucosa of patients with AIDS.

635 ☐ hairy leukoplakia
[héəri lù:koupléikiə]

名 毛状白板症

636 ☐ AIDS
[éidz]

名 エイズ

毛状白板症：エイズ患者の舌や頬粘膜に生じる毛状の表面をもつ白色病変.

---

162. nicotine stomatitis : Heat-stimulated lesions on the palate that begin with erythema and progress to multiple white papules with a red dot in the center, usually caused by habitual pipe smoking.

637 ☐ nicotine stomatitis
[níkəti:n stòumətáitəs]

名 ニコチン性口内炎

ニコチン性口内炎：熱刺激により口蓋に生じる病変. 紅斑に始まり，中央に赤い点をともなう多発性の白い丘疹へと進行する. 通常，習慣的なパイプ喫煙に起因する.

---

163. melanism : Excessive deposition of melanin in the skin.

638 ☐ melanism
[mélənìzm]

名 メラニン沈着

639 ☐ deposition
[dèpəzíʃ(ə)n]

名 沈着

640 ☐ melanin
[mélənən]

名 メラニン

メラニン沈着：皮膚におけるメラニンの過剰な沈着.

9. 口腔粘膜疾患

164. nevus pigmentosus : A pigmented macule or nodule composed of clusters of nevus cells.

641 **nevus pigmentosus**
[níːvəs pìgməntóusəs]

名 **色素性母斑**

642 **nevus**
[níːvəs]

名 **母斑**（複 nevi [níːvài]）

643 **pigmented**
[pígməntid]

形 **色素の沈着した** → pigmentation (525)

> **色素性母斑**：母斑細胞の集塊から成る色素の沈着した斑または小結節．

165. Addison's disease : Chronic adrenocortical insufficiency characterized by fatigue, hypotension, hyperpigmentation, and anorexia.

644 **Addison's disease**
[ǽdəs(ə)nz dizíːz]

名 **アジソン病**

645 **adrenocortical**
[ədrìːnoukɔ́ːrtik(ə)l]

形 **副腎皮質の**

646 **insufficiency**
[ìnsəfíʃ(ə)nsi]

名 **機能低下**

647 **hypotension**
[hàipouténʃ(ə)n]

名 **低血圧**

648 **hyperpigmentation**
[hàipərpìgmənteíʃ(ə)n]

名 **色素沈着過剰** ← pigmentation (525)

649 **anorexia**
[ænəréksiə]

名 **食欲不振**

> **アジソン病**：疲労感，低血圧，色素沈着過剰，食欲不振等を特徴とする慢性の副腎皮質機能低下症．

166. angular stomatitis (=angular cheilitis): Inflammation and fissuring radiating from the angles of the mouth, usually associated with nutritional deficiencies, bacterial or viral infection, mechanical irritation, or atopic dermatitis.

650 **angular stomatitis**
[ǽŋgjələr stòumətáitəs]

名 **口角びらん**

9. 口腔粘膜疾患

651 **angular cheilitis**
[ǽŋgjələr kailáitəs]
名 口角炎

652 **nutritional**
[n(j)utríʃ(ə)n(ə)l]
形 栄養の

653 **deficiency**
[difíʃ(ə)nsi]
名 欠乏

654 **bacterial**
[bæktíəriəl]
形 細菌(性)の ← bacterium (711)

655 **viral**
[váiər(ə)l]
形 ウイルス(性)の ← virus (541)

656 **atopic dermatitis**
[eitápik dɜ̀ːrmətáitəs]
名 アトピー性皮膚炎

657 **dermatitis**
[dɜ̀ːrmətáitəs]
名 皮膚炎

> **口角びらん(＝口角炎)**：口角から広がる炎症および亀裂．通常，栄養欠乏，細菌・ウイルス感染，物理的刺激，アトピー性皮膚炎等に関連する．

167. Plummer-Vinson syndrome：A syndrome usually seen in middle-aged women with iron deficiency anemia, characterized by angular cheilitis, dysphagia, and atrophic glossitis (=bald tongue).

658 **Plummer-Vinson syndrome**
[plʌ́mər vínsən síndròum]
名 プランマー・ヴィンソン症候群

659 **iron deficiency anemia**
[áiərn difíʃ(ə)nsi əníːmiə]
名 鉄欠乏性貧血

660 **atrophic glossitis**
[ətráfik glɑsáitəs]
名 萎縮性舌炎

661 **glossitis**
[glɑsáitəs]
名 舌炎

662 **bald tongue**
[bɔ́ːld tʌ́ŋ]
名 平滑舌

> **プランマー・ヴィンソン症候群**：鉄欠乏性貧血を患う中年女性に好発する症候群．口角炎，嚥下困難，萎縮性舌炎(＝平滑舌)等を特徴とする．

9. 口腔粘膜疾患

168. Hunter's glossitis: Atrophy of the filiform papillae due to vitamin B_{12} deficiencies, resulting in an erythematous, painful tongue with a smooth surface.

663 Hunter's glossitis
[hʌ́ntərz glɑsáitəs]

名 ハンター舌炎

664 filiform papillae
[fíləfɔ̀ːrm pəpíliː]

名 糸状乳頭（複）；（単）〜 papilla [pəpílə]

665 vitamin
[váitəmən]

名 ビタミン

666 erythematous
[èrəθémətəs]

形 紅斑(性)の ← erythema (174)

ハンター舌炎：ビタミン B_{12} 欠乏に起因する糸状乳頭の萎縮．舌の紅斑や疼痛をともない，表面は平滑となる．

---

169. fissured tongue: A tongue with numerous grooves on the dorsal surface.

667 fissured tongue
[fíʃərd tʌ́ŋ]

名 溝状舌

668 dorsal
[dɔ́ːrs(ə)l]

形 背(部)の ← dorsum (671)

溝状舌：背面に多数の溝がある舌．

---

170. black hairy tongue: Black discoloration on the dorsum of the tongue caused by hyperkeratosis of filiform papillae.

669 black hairy tongue
[blǽk héəri tʌ́ŋ]

名 黒毛舌

670 discoloration
[diskʌ̀ləréiʃ(ə)n]

名 変色

671 dorsum
[dɔ́ːrsəm]

名 背(部)

黒毛舌：糸状乳頭の角質増殖に起因する舌の背部の黒い変色．

9. 口腔粘膜疾患

171. geographic tongue：Idiopathic, asymptomatic erythema with a white border on the dorsum of the tongue.

672 □ geographic tongue
[dʒìːəgrǽfik tʌ́ŋ]

|名| 地図状舌

673 □ idiopathic
[ìdiəpǽθik]

|形| 特発性の

> 地図状舌：舌の背部に生じる，白い辺縁をもつ特発性，無症候性の紅斑．

172. median rhomboid glossitis：An asymptomatic, ovoid or rhomboid, erythematous lesion on the median portion of the dorsum of the tongue just anterior to the circumvallate papillae.

674 □ median rhomboid glossitis
[míːdiən rámbɔ̀id glɑsáitəs]

|名| 正中菱形舌炎

675 □ circumvallate papillae
[sə̀ːrkəmvǽlèit pəpíliː]

|名| 有郭乳頭（複；単 ～ papilla [pəpílə]）

> 正中菱形舌炎：舌の背部中央，有郭乳頭の前方に生じる，無症候性で，卵形または菱形の紅斑性病変．

173. Fordyce spots：Ectopic sebaceous glands in the oral mucosa that appear as numerous yellowish-white spots.

676 □ Fordyce spots
[fɔ́ːrdàis spʌ́ts]

|名| フォーダイス斑

> フォーダイス斑：口腔粘膜内の異所性脂腺．多数の黄白色の斑点として観察される．

174. lingual tonsil hypertrophy：Abnormal enlargement of the lingual tonsil due to inflammation or mechanical stimulation.

677 □ lingual tonsil hypertrophy
[líŋwəl táns(ə)l haipə́ːrtrəfi]

|名| 舌扁桃肥大

9. 口腔粘膜疾患

678 lingual tonsil
[líŋwəl táns(ə)l]

名 舌扁桃

舌扁桃肥大：炎症や物理的刺激に起因する舌扁桃の異常な肥大．

175. cheilitis：Inflammation of the lips that affects the labial mucosa, the vermilion border, and the perioral skin.

679 cheilitis
[kailáitəs]

名 口唇炎

680 labial mucosa
[léibiəl mjukóusə]

名 口唇粘膜

681 vermilion border
[vərmíljən bɔ́:rdər]

名 赤唇縁

口唇炎：口唇粘膜，赤唇縁，口周囲の皮膚等に及ぶ口唇の炎症．

176. granulomatous cheilitis：Chronic, diffuse swelling of the lips characterized by noncaseating epithelioid cell granulomas in the dermis.

682 granulomatous cheilitis
[grænjəlóumətəs kailáitəs]

名 肉芽腫性口唇炎

683 noncaseating
[nɑnkéisièitiŋ]

形 非乾酪性の

684 epithelioid cell
[èpəθí:liòid sél]

名 類上皮細胞

685 dermis
[dɔ́:rməs]

名 真皮

肉芽腫性口唇炎：口唇の慢性，びまん性の腫脹で，真皮内の非乾酪性類上皮細胞肉芽腫を特徴とする．

177. Melkersson-Rosenthal syndrome：A syndrome characterized by granulomatous cheilitis, paralysis of the facial nerve, and fissured tongue.

686 Melkersson-Rosenthal syndrome
[mélkərs(ə)n róuzənta:l síndròum]

名 メルカーソン・ローゼンタール症候群

9. 口腔粘膜疾患

687 **paralysis**
[pərǽləsəs]

名 麻痺

688 **facial nerve**
[féiʃ(ə)l nə́ːrv]

名 顔面神経

> メルカーソン・ローゼンタール症候群：肉芽腫性口唇炎，顔面神経麻痺，溝状舌を特徴とする症候群．

178. contact cheilitis : Acute inflammation of the lips resulting from contact with an irritant or allergen.

689 **contact cheilitis**
[kántækt kailáitəs]

名 接触性口唇炎

690 **irritant**
[írətənt]

名 刺激性物質

691 **allergen**
[ǽlərdʒèn]

名 アレルゲン

> 接触性口唇炎：刺激性物質やアレルゲンとの接触に起因する急性の口唇炎．

179. Riga-Fede disease : Ulceration of the lingual frenulum in teething infants, associated with abrasion of the tissue against central incisors.

692 **Riga-Fede disease**
[ríːɡɑː féidei dizíːz]

名 リガ・フェーデ病

693 **ulceration**
[ʌ̀lsəréiʃ(ə)n]

名 潰瘍化 ← ulcer (538)

694 **teethe**
[tíːð]

動 歯が生える

695 **infant**
[ínfənt]

名 乳児

696 **abrasion**
[əbréiʒ(ə)n]

名 擦過傷

> リガ・フェーデ病：歯生期の乳児に見られる舌小帯の潰瘍化．中切歯による組織への擦過傷に関連する．

9. 口腔粘膜疾患

180. Bednar's aphthae: Traumatic ulcers located bilaterally on either side of the midpalatal raphe in infants.

697 **Bednar's aphthae** [bédnɑːrz ǽfθiː]

名 **ベドナー・アフタ**（複；単 ～ aphtha [ǽfθə]）

698 aphtha [ǽfθə]

名 **アフタ**（複 aphthae [ǽfθiː]）

699 traumatic [trɔːmǽtik]

形 **外傷（性）の** ← trauma (64)

700 midpalatal [mìdpǽlət(ə)l]

形 **口蓋中央の**

701 raphe [réifi]

名 **縫線**

> ベドナー・アフタ：乳児の口蓋の正中縫線の両側に見られる外傷性の潰瘍.

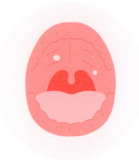

10 骨の疾患

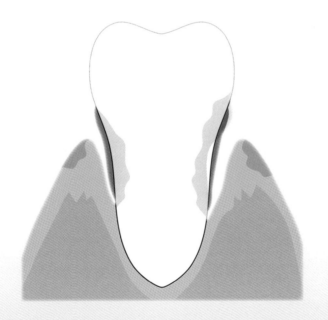

10. 骨の疾患

181. alveolar osteitis: Inflammation of the alveolar bone associated with apical periodontitis or infection after tooth extraction.

702 **alveolar osteitis** [ælvíːələr àstiáitəs]
名 歯槽骨炎

703 **osteitis** [àstiáitəs]
名 骨炎

歯槽骨炎：根尖性歯周炎や抜歯後の感染に関連する歯槽骨の炎症．

---

182. periostitis: Inflammation of the periosteum due to acute or chronic infection or trauma, characterized by tenderness and swelling of the affected site, fever, and chills.

704 **periostitis** [pèriəstáitəs]
名 骨膜炎

705 **periosteum** [pèriástiəm]
名 骨膜

706 **tenderness** [téndərnəs]
名 圧痛

707 **chill** [tʃíl]
名 悪寒

骨膜炎：急性・慢性の感染症や外傷に起因する骨膜の炎症．患部の圧痛および腫脹，発熱，悪寒等を特徴とする．

---

183. osteomyelitis: Inflammation of the bone and bone marrow due to pyogenic bacteria, characterized by localized pain and tenderness with or without constitutional symptoms.

708 **osteomyelitis** [àstioumàiəláitəs]
名 骨髄炎

709 **bone marrow** [bóun mǽrou]
名 骨髄

710 **pyogenic** [pàioudʒénik]
形 化膿性の

711 **bacteria** [bæktíəriə]
名 細菌 （複；単 bacterium [bæktíəriəm]）

10. 骨の疾患

⁷¹² constitutional symptom
[kànstət(j)úːʃ(ə)n(ə)l símptəm]

【名】全身症状

骨髄炎：化膿菌に起因する骨および骨髄の炎症．限局性の疼痛・圧痛を特徴とし，全身症状をともなうこともある．

184. bisphosphonate-related osteonecrosis of the jaw (BRONJ)：A side effect of bisphosphonate that causes osteonecrosis of the jaw in a person who undergoes dental surgery.

⁷¹³ bisphosphonate-related osteonecrosis of the jaw (BRONJ)
[bisfásfənèit riléitid àstiounekróusəs əv ðə dʒɔ́ː]

【名】ビスフォスフォネート関連顎骨壊死

⁷¹⁴ bisphosphonate
[bisfásfənèit]

【名】ビスフォスフォネート

⁷¹⁵ osteonecrosis
[àstiounekróusəs]

【名】骨壊死

⁷¹⁶ side effect
[sáid ifékt]

【名】副作用

ビスフォスフォネート関連顎骨壊死：ビスフォスフォネートの副作用で，歯の外科的処置を受けた患者に顎骨壊死を生じさせる．

11 顎関節疾患

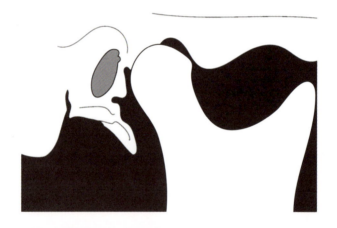

11. 顎関節疾患

185. mandibular condylar hyperplasia: Overdevelopment of the mandibular condyle, unilaterally or bilaterally, leading to facial asymmetry and malocclusion.

717 □ mandibular condylar hyperplasia
[mændíbjələr kándələr hàipərpléiʒ(i)ə]

名 下顎頭過形成

718 □ mandibular condyle
[mændíbjələr kándàil]

名 下顎頭，顆頭

719 □ facial asymmetry
[féiʃ(ə)l eisímətri]

名 顔面非対称

> **下顎頭過形成**：下顎頭の片側性または両側性の過成長．顔面非対称や不正咬合の原因となる．

186. temporomandibular joint disorder: Noninflammatory dysfunction of temporomandibular joint characterized by pain, cracking, and limited mandibular opening.

720 □ temporomandibular joint disorder
[tèmpəroumændíbjələr dʒɔ́int disɔ́:rdər]

名 顎関節症

721 □ temporomandibular joint
[tèmpəroumændíbjələr dʒɔ́int]

名 顎関節

722 □ joint
[dʒɔ́int]

名 関節

> **顎関節症**：顎関節の非炎症性機能障害．疼痛，軋音，下顎の開口制限等を特徴とする．

187. osteoarthritis: A progressive joint disease characterized by degeneration of the articular cartilage, proliferation of osteophytes, and inflammation of the synovial membrane.

723 □ osteoarthritis
[àstiouɑ:rθráitəs]

名 変形性関節症

724 □ articular
[ɑ:rtíkjələr]

形 関節の

11. 顎関節疾患

725 ☐ **articular cartilage**
[ɑːrtíkjələr kɑ́ːrtəlidʒ]
名 関節軟骨

726 ☐ **cartilage**
[kɑ́ːrtəlidʒ]
名 軟骨

727 ☐ **osteophyte**
[ɑ́stiəfàit]
名 骨棘

728 ☐ **synovial**
[sənóuviəl]
形 滑膜の

729 ☐ **synovial membrane**
[sənóuviəl mémbrèin]
名 滑膜

> **変形性関節症**：関節軟骨の変性，骨棘の増殖，滑膜の炎症等を特徴とする進行性の関節疾患．

188. traumatic arthritis: An acute or chronic inflammation of a joint as a result of injury.

730 ☐ **traumatic arthritis**
[trɔːmǽtik ɑːrθráitəs]
名 外傷性関節炎

> **外傷性関節炎**：外傷に起因する関節の急性または慢性の炎症．

189. suppurative arthritis: Bacterial infection of synovial or periarticular tissues, accompanied by arthralgia, stiffness, and purulent effusion.

731 ☐ **suppurative arthritis**
[sʌ́pjərèitiv ɑːrθráitəs]
名 化膿性関節炎

732 ☐ **periarticular**
[pèriɑːrtíkjələr]
形 関節周囲の ← articular (724)

733 ☐ **stiffness**
[stífnəs]
名 硬直

734 ☐ **purulent**
[pjúərələnt]
形 化膿性の

735 ☐ **effusion**
[ifjúːʒ(ə)n]
名 滲出

> **化膿性関節炎**：細菌による滑膜組織または関節周囲組織の感染症．関節痛，硬直，化膿性浸出等をともなう．

11. 顎関節疾患

190. Costen syndrome: A syndrome characterized by temporomandibular joint dysfunction, hearing loss, tinnitus, burning pain of the throat, and headache.

736	Costen syndrome [kást(ə)n síndròum]	名 コステン症候群
737	hearing loss [híəriŋ lɔ́s]	名 難聴
738	tinnitus [tənáitəs]	名 耳鳴り
739	burning pain [bə́ːrniŋ péin]	名 灼熱痛

コステン症候群：顎関節の機能障害，難聴，耳鳴り，咽頭部灼熱痛，頭痛等を特徴とする症候群．

---

191. rheumatoid arthritis: A chronic autoimmune disease that causes inflammation and deformity of the joints.

740	rheumatoid arthritis [rúːmətɔ̀id ɑːrθráitəs]	名 関節リウマチ
741	deformity [difɔ́ːrməti]	名 変形

関節リウマチ：関節の炎症と変形を生じる慢性の自己免疫疾患．

---

192. gout: A disorder of purine metabolism characterized by hyperuricemia and recurrent acute arthritis resulting from deposition of sodium urate crystals in connective tissues and articular cartilage.

742	gout [gáut]	名 痛風
743	purine [pjúəriːn]	名 プリン
744	metabolism [mətǽbəlizm]	名 代謝
745	hyperuricemia [hàipərjùərəsíːmiə]	名 高尿酸血症

11. 顎関節疾患

746 **sodium urate**
[sóudiəm júərèit]

名 尿酸ナトリウム

747 **crystal**
[kríst(ə)l]

名 結晶

> **痛風**：高尿酸血症と尿酸ナトリウム結晶の結合組織および関節軟骨への沈着に起因する再発性の急性関節炎を特徴とするプリン代謝異常．

193. articular chondrocalcinosis：A disease characterized by deposition of calcium pyrophosphate crystals in synovial fluid, articular cartilage, and adjacent soft tissue, causing swelling of joints and goutlike painful attacks.

748 **articular chondrocalcinosis**
[ɑːrtíkjələr kàndroukælsənóusəs]

名 関節軟骨石灰化症

749 **chondrocalcinosis**
[kàndroukælsənóusəs]

名 軟骨石灰化(症)

750 **calcium pyrophosphate**
[kælsiəm pàiəroufásfèit]

名 ピロリン酸カルシウム

751 **synovial fluid**
[sənóuviəl flúːəd]

名 滑液

> **関節軟骨石灰化症**：滑液，関節軟骨，および周囲の軟組織におけるピロリン酸カルシウム結晶の沈着を特徴とする疾患．関節の腫脹と痛風様の疼痛発作を生じる．

194. osteochondroma：A benign bone tumor occurring most commonly at the ends of long bones.

752 **osteochondroma**
[àstioukɑndróumə]

名 骨軟骨腫

> **骨軟骨腫**：長骨の骨端部に好発する良性の骨腫瘍．

11. 顎関節疾患

195. synovial chondromatosis: A tumorlike bone lesion characterized by numerous calcified cartilaginous bodies in the synovial membrane.

753 **synovial chondromatosis**
[sənóuviəl kɑndròumətóusəs]

名 滑膜軟骨腫症

754 **chondromatosis**
[kɑndròumətóusəs]

名 軟骨腫(症)

755 **cartilaginous**
[kɑ̀:rtəlǽdʒənəs]

形 軟骨(性)の ← cartilage (726)

滑膜軟骨腫症：滑膜中に多数の石灰化した軟骨塊を生じる骨の腫瘍類似病変．

---

196. ankylosis: Fixation and immobility of a joint as a result of disease or trauma.

756 **ankylosis**
[æ̀ŋkilóusəs]

名 関節強直

関節強直：疾患または外傷に起因する関節の癒着および可動性喪失．

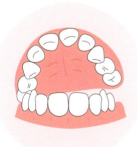

12 | 唾液腺疾患

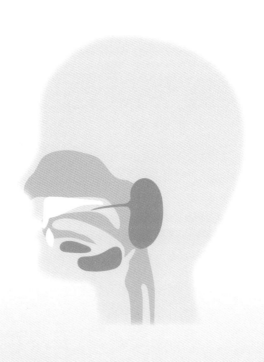

12. 唾液腺疾患

197. <u>accessory salivary gland</u>：Ectopic salivary gland tissue with a duct system.

757 □ <u>accessory salivary gland</u>
[æksésəri sǽləvèri glǽnd]

名 副唾液腺

副唾液腺：異所性の唾液腺組織で導管系を有する．

198. <u>aberrant salivary gland</u>：Ectopic salivary gland tissue without any duct system.

758 □ <u>aberrant salivary gland</u>
[æbérənt sǽləvèri glǽnd]

名 迷入唾液腺

迷入唾液腺：異所性の唾液腺組織で導管系をもたない．

199. <u>salivary fistula</u>：An abnormal passage from a salivary gland or duct to an opening in the mouth or on the skin of the face or neck.

759 □ <u>salivary fistula</u>
[sǽləvèri fístʃələ]

名 唾液瘻

唾液瘻：唾液腺や導管から口腔内または顔面・頸部皮膚上の開口部へ通じる異常な通路．

200. <u>xerostomia (=dry mouth)</u>：Abnormal dryness of the mouth due to reduced secretion of saliva.

760 □ <u>xerostomia</u>
[zìəroustóumiə]

名 口腔乾燥症

761 □ <u>dry mouth</u>
[drái máuθ]

名 ドライマウス

762 □ <u>secretion</u>
[sikríːʃ(ə)n]

名 分泌

763 □ <u>saliva</u>
[səláivə]

名 唾液

口腔乾燥症(＝ドライマウス)：唾液の分泌減少に起因する口腔内の異常な乾燥．

12. 唾液腺疾患

201. **sialorrhea**：Excessive secretion of saliva.

764 □ sialorrhea
[sàiələrí:ə]

名 流涎症

流涎症：唾液の過剰分泌．

202. **sialadenitis**：Bacterial infection of a salivary gland, usually due to a sialolith or gland hyposecretion.

765 □ sialadenitis
[sàiəlǽdənáitəs]

名 唾液腺炎

766 □ sialolith
[saiǽlouliθ]

名 唾石

767 □ hyposecretion
[hàipousikrí:ʃ(ə)n]

名 分泌不全　← secretion (762)

唾液腺炎：細菌による唾液腺の感染症で，通常，唾石または腺の分泌不全に起因する．

203. **sialoangiitis**：Inflammation of salivary gland ducts, usually associated with sialadenitis.

768 □ sialoangiitis
[sàiəlouændʒiáitəs]

名 唾液管炎

唾液管炎：唾液腺導管の炎症で，通常，唾液腺炎にともなって生じる．

204. **epidemic parotitis (=mumps)**：An acute contagious disease caused by a paramyxovirus and characterized by inflammation and swelling of the salivary glands, especially the parotid glands.

769 □ epidemic parotitis
[èpədémik pærətáitəs]

名 流行性耳下腺炎

770 □ mumps
[mʌ́mps]

名 おたふくかぜ

771 □ epidemic
[èpədémik]

形 流行性の　**名** 流行

772 □ contagious
[kəntéidʒəs]

形 伝染性の

12. 唾液腺疾患

773 ☐ **paramyxovirus**
[pæ̀rəmíksəvàiərəs]

名 パラミクソウイルス

流行性耳下腺炎（＝おたふくかぜ）：パラミクソウイルスによる急性伝染性疾患で，唾液腺，とくに耳下腺の炎症と腫脹を特徴とする．

---

205. Mikulicz disease: An autoimmune disease characterized by bilateral painless enlargement of the lacrimal and salivary glands.

774 ☐ **Mikulicz disease**
[mí:kulìtʃ dizí:z]

名 ミクリッツ病

ミクリッツ病：涙腺と唾液腺の両側性・無痛性腫脹を特徴とする自己免疫疾患．

---

206. Sjögren syndrome: A chronic autoimmune disease occurring mostly in middle-aged women, characterized by keratoconjunctivitis sicca, xerostomia, rheumatoid arthritis, and enlargement of the parotid glands.

775 ☐ **Sjögren syndrome**
[ʃɔ́:grèn síndròum]

名 シェーグレン症候群

776 ☐ **keratoconjunctivitis**
[kèrətoukəndʒʌ̀ŋktiváitəs]

名 角結膜炎

777 ☐ **keratoconjunctivitis sicca**
[kèrətoukəndʒʌ̀ŋktiváitəs síkə]

名 乾性角結膜炎

シェーグレン症候群：中年期の女性に好発する慢性の自己免疫疾患で，乾性角結膜炎，口腔乾燥症，関節リウマチ，耳下腺の腫脹等を特徴とする．

---

207. Frey syndrome: Localized flushing and sweating of the ear and cheek in response to eating, due to damage of the parasympathetic fibers in the auriculotemporal nerve.

778 ☐ **Frey syndrome**
[fréi síndròum]

名 フライ症候群

779 ☐ **flushing**
[flʌ́ʃiŋ]

名 紅潮

780 ☐ **sweating**
[swétiŋ]

名 発汗

12. 唾液腺疾患

781 parasympathetic
[pæ̀rəsìmpəθétik]

形 副交感神経の ↔ sympathetic (999)

782 auriculotemporal nerve
[ɔːrìkjəloutémpər(ə)l nə́ːrv]

名 耳介側頭神経

フライ症候群：食事にともなう耳や頬の限局性紅潮および発汗．耳介側頭神経の副交感神経線維の損傷に起因する．

208. sialolithiasis：A pathological condition in which calculi are formed in a salivary gland duct.

783 sialolithiasis
[sàiəlouliθáiəsəs]

名 唾石症

784 pathological
[pæ̀θəládʒik(ə)l]

形 病的な，病理学（上）の

785 calculi
[kǽlkjəlài]

名 結石（複；単 calculus [kǽlkjələs]）

唾石症：唾液腺導管内に結石を生じる病態．

209. necrotizing sialometaplasia：Squamous cell metaplasia of the salivary gland ducts and lobules associated with necrosis of the gland tissue.

786 necrotizing sialometaplasia
[nékrətàizin sàiəloumètəpléiʒ(i)ə]

名 壊死性唾液腺化生

787 sialometaplasia
[sàiəloumètəpléiʒ(i)ə]

名 唾液腺化生

788 metaplasia
[mètəpléiʒ(i)ə]

名 化生

789 lobule
[lábjul]

名 小葉

壊死性唾液腺化生：唾液腺導管および小葉の扁平上皮化生で，腺組織の壊死に関連する．

13 神経疾患

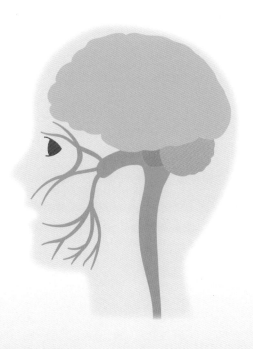

13. 神経疾患

210. trigeminal neuralgia: Severe paroxysmal pain in one or more branches of the trigeminal nerve, induced by chewing, talking, or stimulating trigger points in or about the mouth.

#	英語	品詞	日本語
790	trigeminal neuralgia [traidʒémən(ə)l n(j)uərǽldʒ(i)ə]	名	三叉神経痛
791	neuralgia [n(j)uərǽldʒ(i)ə]	名	神経痛
792	paroxysmal [pæ̀rəksízm(ə)l]	形	発作(性)の
793	trigeminal nerve [traidʒémən(ə)l nə́ːrv]	名	三叉神経
794	chewing [tʃúːiŋ]	名	咀嚼
795	trigger point [trígər pɔ́int]	名	発痛点

三叉神経痛：1本以上の三叉神経枝に生じる激しい発作性疼痛．咀嚼，会話，口内あるいは口付近の発痛点への刺激等により誘発される．

---

210. glossopharyngeal neuralgia: Severe paroxysmal pain in the glossopharyngeal nerve distribution (posterior pharynx, tonsils, root of the tongue), induced by chewing, swallowing, talking, or yawning.

#	英語	品詞	日本語
796	glossopharyngeal neuralgia [glɑ̀soufæ̀rəndʒíːəl n(j)uərǽldʒ(i)ə]	名	舌咽神経痛
797	glossopharyngeal nerve [glɑ̀soufæ̀rəndʒíːəl nə́ːrv]	名	舌咽神経
798	pharynx [fǽriŋks]	名	咽頭
799	root of tongue [rúːt əv tʌ́ŋ]	名	舌根
800	swallowing [swɑ́louiŋ]	名	嚥下

舌咽神経痛：舌咽神経の分布領域（咽頭後部，扁桃，舌根）に生じる激しい発作性疼痛．咀嚼，嚥下，会話，あくび等により誘発される．

13. 神経疾患

212. complex regional pain syndrome (CRPS): Chronic neuropathic pain that usually follows injury, accompanied by edema, limited joint motion, and atrophic changes of the skin.

801 complex regional pain syndrome (CRPS)
[kámplèks ríːdʒən(ə)l péin síndròum]
名 複合性局所疼痛症候群

802 neuropathic
[n(j)ùəroupǽθik]
形 神経障害性の

> 複合性局所疼痛症候群：通常，外傷後に発症する慢性の神経障害性疼痛で，浮腫，関節の運動制限，皮膚の萎縮性変化等をともなう．

213. glossodynia: An idiopathic syndrome of pain in the tongue without apparent lesions, often associated with ageusia.

803 glossodynia
[glàsoudíniə]
名 舌痛症

804 ageusia
[əgjúːziə]
名 味覚消失

> 舌痛症：明らかな病変は認められないが舌に疼痛を生じる特発性症候群で，しばしば味覚消失をともなう．

214. facial paralysis: Paresis or paralysis of the facial muscles due to either a lesion involving either the nucleus or the facial nerve peripheral to the nucleus (peripheral paralysis) or a supranuclear lesion in the cerebrum or upper brainstem (central paralysis).

805 facial paralysis
[féiʃ(ə)l pərǽləsəs]
名 顔面神経麻痺

806 paresis
[pəríːsəs]
名 不全麻痺

807 facial muscles
[féiʃ(ə)l mʌ́s(ə)lz]
名 顔面筋，表情筋（複；通常は複数形を使用する）

808 nucleus
[n(j)úːkliəs]
名 核，神経核

809 peripheral
[pərífər(ə)l]
形 末梢(性)の

13. 神経疾患

810 supranuclear
[sùːprən(j)úːkliər]

形 核上(性)の ← nucleus (808)

811 cerebrum
[səríːbrəm]

名 大脳

812 brainstem
[bréinstèm]

名 脳幹

> **顔面神経麻痺**：顔面筋の不全麻痺または麻痺．核または核より末梢の顔面神経の病変による末梢性麻痺と，大脳または脳幹上部の核上性病変による中枢性麻痺に分けられる．

215. Ramsay Hunt syndrome：Reactivation of the herpes zoster virus in the geniculate ganglion, characterized by facial paralysis, tinnitus, hearing loss, vertigo, and vesicles in the ear canal.

813 Ramsay Hunt syndrome
[rǽmsi hǎnt síndròum]

名 ラムゼイ・ハント症候群

814 geniculate ganglion
[dʒəníkjələt gǽŋgliən]

名 膝神経節

815 ganglion
[gǽŋgliən]

名 神経節

816 vertigo
[vɚ́ːrtigòu]

名 めまい

817 ear canal
[íər kənǽl]

名 外耳道

> **ラムゼイ・ハント症候群**：帯状疱疹ウイルスの膝神経節における再活性化で，顔面神経麻痺，耳鳴り，難聴，めまい，外耳道の小水疱等を特徴とする．

216. Bell's palsy：Idiopathic peripheral facial paralysis.

818 Bell's palsy
[bélz pɔ́ːlzi]

名 ベル麻痺

819 palsy
[pɔ́ːlzi]

名 麻痺（主に合成語で用いられる）

> **ベル麻痺**：特発性の末梢性顔面神経麻痺．

13. 神経疾患

217. facial spasm：Unilateral involuntary contractions of facial muscles due to dysfunction of the seventh cranial nerve or its motor nucleus.

820 □ facial spasm
[féiʃ(ə)l spǽzm]
名 顔面痙攣

821 □ spasm
[spǽzm]
名 痙攣

822 □ involuntary
[inváləntèri]
形 不随意の

823 □ contraction
[kəntrǽkʃ(ə)n]
名 収縮

824 □ cranial nerve
[kréiniəl nə́ːrv]
名 脳神経

825 □ motor nucleus
[móutər n(j)úːkliəs]
名 運動核

顔面痙攣：第七脳神経またはその運動核の機能障害に起因する顔面筋の片側性不随意収縮．

---

218. oral dyskinesia：Involuntary movements of the lips and tongue that develop mostly as a delayed complication of antipsychotic agents.

826 □ oral dyskinesia
[ɔ́ːr(ə)l dìskəníːʒ(i)ə]
名 口腔ジスキネジア

827 □ dyskinesia
[dìskəníːʒ(i)ə]
名 ジスキネジア

828 □ antipsychotic agent
[æ̀ntisaikátik éidʒənt]
名 抗精神病薬

口腔ジスキネジア：主に抗精神病薬の遅発合併症として生じる口唇や舌の不随意運動．

13. 神経疾患

219. dysgeusia: Unpleasant alteration of the sense of taste or decrease in taste sensitivity.

829 □ <u>dysgeusia</u>
[disgjúːʒ(i)ə]

830 □ sense of taste
[séns əv téist]

831 □ sensitivity
[sènsətívəti]

名 味覚異常

名 味覚

名 感受性

味覚異常：味覚の不快な変化または味の感受性の低下．

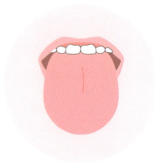

14 歯・口腔・顎顔面に異常を来す疾患・症候群

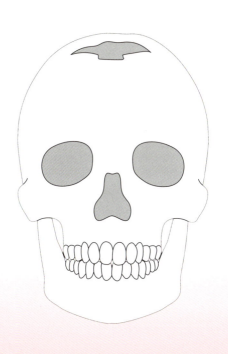

14. 歯・口腔・顎顔面に異常を来す疾患・症候群

220. cleidocranial dysplasia (=cleidocranial dysostosis)：A hereditary disorder characterized by absence or hypoplasia of clavicles, defective ossification of the cranium, and malocclusion.

832 □ **cleidocranial dysplasia** [klàidoukréiniəl displéiʒ(i)ə]
名 鎖骨頭蓋異形成症

833 □ **cleidocranial dysostosis** [klàidoukréiniəl dìsastóusəs]
名 鎖骨頭蓋異骨症

834 □ **dysostosis** [dìsastóusəs]
名 異骨症

835 □ **clavicle** [klǽvək(ə)l]
名 鎖骨

836 □ **ossification** [àsəfəkéiʃ(ə)n]
名 骨化

837 □ **cranium** [kréiniəm]
名 頭蓋 = skull (915)

鎖骨頭蓋異形成症(＝鎖骨頭蓋異骨症)：鎖骨の欠損または形成不全，頭蓋の骨化障害，不正咬合等を特徴とする遺伝性疾患．

221. osteopetrosis (=marble bone disease)：A hereditary disorder characterized by a generalized increase in bone density caused by faulty bone resorption resulting from dysfunction of osteoclasts.

838 □ **osteopetrosis** [àstioupətróusəs]
名 大理石骨病

839 □ **marble bone disease** [máːrbl bóun dizíːz]
名 大理石骨病

840 □ **generalized** [dʒénərəlàizd]
形 全身(性)の ↔ localized (113)

841 □ **bone density** [bóun dénsəti]
名 骨密度

842 □ **bone resorption** [bóun risɔ́ːrpʃ(ə)n]
名 骨吸収

843 □ **osteoclast** [ástiəklæst]
名 破骨細胞

大理石骨病：全身性の骨密度上昇を特徴とする遺伝性疾患．破骨細胞の機能不全による骨吸収障害に起因する．

14. 歯・口腔・顎顔面に異常を来す疾患・症候群

222. osteogenesis imperfecta: A hereditary collagen disorder characterized by bone fragility, blue sclera, joint laxity, and hearing loss.

844	osteogenesis imperfecta [ùstioudʒénəsəs ìmpərféktə]	名 骨形成不全症
845	collagen [kάlədʒən]	名 コラーゲン
846	fragility [frədʒíləti]	名 脆弱性
847	sclera [sklíərə]	名 強膜
848	joint laxity [dʒɔ́int lǽksəti]	名 関節弛緩

<u>骨形成不全症</u>：骨脆弱性，青色強膜，関節弛緩，難聴等を特徴とする遺伝性のコラーゲン異常．

223. Treacher Collins syndrome (=mandibulofacial dysostosis): Defective bone formation of the face and lower jaw characterized by downwardly slanting palpebral fissures, coloboma of the lower eyelid, malformed auricle, and hearing loss.

849	Treacher Collins syndrome [tríːtʃər kάlənz síndròum]	名 トリーチャー・コリンズ症候群
850	mandibulofacial dysostosis [mændìbjəlouféiʃ(ə)l dìsαstóusəs]	名 下顎顔面異骨症
851	palpebral [pælpíːbr(ə)l]	形 眼瞼の ← palpebra (1000)
852	palpebral fissure [pælpíːbr(ə)l fíʃər]	名 眼瞼裂
853	coloboma [kὰləbóumə]	名 欠損
854	eyelid [áilìd]	名 眼瞼 = palpebra (1000)
855	auricle [ɔ́ːrik(ə)l]	名 耳介

14. 歯・口腔・顎顔面に異常を来す疾患・症候群

> **トリーチャー・コリンズ症候群（＝下顎顔面異骨症）**：眼瞼裂の下方傾斜，下眼瞼の欠損，耳介の奇形，難聴等を特徴とする顔面と下顎の骨形成不全．

224. Crouzon syndrome (=craniofacial dysostosis)：Craniosynostosis with broad forehead, hypertelorism, exophthalmos, beak-like nose, and hypoplasia of the maxilla.

856 **Crouzon syndrome** [kruzán síndròum] — 名 クルーゾン症候群

857 **craniofacial dysostosis** [krèiniouféiʃ(ə)l dìsastóusəs] — 名 頭蓋顔面異骨症

858 **craniosynostosis** [krèiniousìnastóusəs] — 名 頭蓋縫合早期癒合症

859 **hypertelorism** [hàipərtélərìzm] — 名 両眼隔離

860 **exophthalmos** [èksafθǽlmàs] — 名 眼球突出

> **クルーゾン症候群（＝頭蓋顔面異骨症）**：広い額，両眼隔離，眼球突出，くちばしに似た鼻，上顎骨の形成不全等をともなう頭蓋縫合早期癒合症．

225. Apert syndrome (=acrocephalosyndactyly)：Craniosynostosis with partial or complete fusion of the fingers and toes.

861 **Apert syndrome** [ɑːpéər síndròum] — 名 アペール症候群

862 **acrocephalosyndactyly** [ækrousèfəlousindǽktəli] — 名 尖頭合指症

> **アペール症候群（＝尖頭合指症）**：手指・足指の一部または完全な癒合をともなう頭蓋縫合早期癒合症．

226. achondroplasia：A congenital disorder of cartilage formation leading to short-limb dwarfism, characterized by a large head with frontal bossing, saddle nose, lumbar lordosis, and genu varum.

863 **achondroplasia** [èikàndroupléiʒ(i)ə] — 名 軟骨無形成症

14. 歯・口腔・顎顔面に異常を来す疾患・症候群

864 limb
[lím]
名 肢

865 dwarfism
[dwɔ́ːrfizm]
名 低身長症

866 frontal bossing
[fránt(ə)l básiŋ]
名 前頭隆起

867 saddle nose
[sǽdl nóuz]
名 鞍鼻

868 lumbar
[lámbər]
形 腰の，腰椎の

869 lordosis
[lɔːrdóusəs]
名 前彎

870 genu varum
[dʒíːnùː véirəm]
名 内反膝

軟骨無形成症：四肢短縮型低身長症の原因となる先天性の軟骨形成異常．前頭隆起をともなう大きな頭，鞍鼻，腰椎前彎，内反膝等を特徴とする．

227. first and second branchial arch syndrome：A congenital disorder caused by a failure of neural crest cells to migrate into the first and second branchial arches, characterized by facial asymmetry, malformed auricle, and mandibular hypoplasia.

871 first and second branchial arch syndrome
[fə́ːrst ənd sékənd brǽŋkiəl áːrtʃ síndròum]
名 第一第二鰓弓症候群

872 branchial arch
[brǽŋkiəl áːrtʃ]
名 鰓弓

873 neural crest
[n(j)úər(ə)l krést]
名 神経堤

874 migrate
[máigrèit]
動 遊走する

第一第二鰓弓症候群：神経堤細胞の第一第二鰓弓への遊走異常に起因する先天性疾患．顔面非対称，耳介の奇形，下顎形成不全等を特徴とする．

14. 歯・口腔・顎顔面に異常を来す疾患・症候群

228. <u>Goldenhar syndrome</u>：A congenital disorder associated with anomalous development of the first and second branchial arches and characterized by epibulbar lipodermoid, preauricular tags, micrognathia, and vertebral malformation.

875 <u>Goldenhar syndrome</u> [góuldənhà:r síndròum] — 名 ゴールデンハー症候群

876 epibulbar [èpəbʌ́lbər] — 形 眼球上の

877 lipodermoid [lìpoudə́:rmòid] — 名 脂肪類皮腫

878 preauricular [pri:ɔ:ríkjələr] — 形 耳介前方の ← auricle (855)

879 micrognathia [màikrounéiθiə] — 名 小顎症

880 vertebral [və́:rtəbr(ə)l] — 形 脊柱の ← vertebra (378)

> ゴールデンハー症候群：第一第二鰓弓の発育異常に関連する先天性疾患．眼球上の脂肪類皮腫，耳介前方の突起物，小顎症，脊柱の奇形等を特徴とする．

229. <u>oral-facial-digital syndrome</u>：An autosomal recessive or X-linked syndrome with varying combinations of defects of the oral cavity, face, and hands, including lobulated or bifid tongue, cleft palate, tongue tumors, missing or malposed teeth, hypoplastic alar cartilage, depressed nasal bridge, brachydactyly, and clinodactyly.

881 <u>oral-facial-digital syndrome</u> [ɔ́:r(ə)l féiʃ(ə)l dídʒət(ə)l síndròum] — 名 口腔顔面指趾症候群

882 autosomal [ɔ̀:təsóuməl] — 形 常染色体(性)の

883 recessive [risésiv] — 形 劣性の ↔ dominant (902)

884 X-linked [éks líŋkt] — 形 X連鎖の

885 lobulated tongue [lábjəlèitid tʌ́ŋ] — 名 分葉舌

886 bifid tongue [báifid tʌ́ŋ] — 名 二裂舌

14. 歯・口腔・顎顔面に異常を来す疾患・症候群

887 □ **malposed** [mælpóuzd] — 形 位置異常の

888 □ **hypoplastic** [hàipouplǽstik] — 形 形成不全の ← hypoplasia (52)

889 □ **alar cartilage** [éilər káːrtəlidʒ] — 名 鼻翼軟骨

890 □ **nasal bridge** [néiz(ə)l brídʒ] — 名 鼻梁

891 □ **brachydactyly** [brækidǽktəli] — 名 短指

892 □ **clinodactyly** [klàinoudǽktəli] — 名 斜指

> **口腔顔面指趾症候群**：口腔，顔面，手の奇形が種々に組み合わさった常染色体劣性遺伝または X 連鎖遺伝による症候群．分葉舌または二裂舌，口蓋裂，舌腫瘍，歯の欠損または位置異常，鼻翼軟骨の形成不全，鼻梁の陥没，短指，斜指等をともなう．

230. Marfan syndrome

A multisystemic connective tissue disorder characterized by skeletal changes (arachnodactyly, long limbs, joint laxity), cardiovascular defects (aortic dissection, mitral valve prolapse), and ectopia lentis.

893 □ **Marfan syndrome** [máːrfæn síndròum] — 名 マルファン症候群

894 □ **multisystemic** [mÀltisistémik] — 形 多系統(性)の

895 □ **arachnodactyly** [əræknoudǽktəli] — 名 クモ指

896 □ **cardiovascular** [kàːrdiouvǽskjələr] — 形 心血管の

897 □ **aortic dissection** [eióːrtik disékʃ(ə)n] — 名 大動脈解離

898 □ **mitral valve prolapse** [máitr(ə)l vælv proulǽps] — 名 僧房弁逸脱

899 □ **ectopia lentis** [ektóupiə léntəs] — 名 水晶体偏位

> **マルファン症候群**：骨格変化(クモ指，長い四肢，関節弛緩)，心血管障害(大動脈解離，僧房弁逸脱)，水晶体偏位等を特徴とする多系統性の結合組織疾患．

14. 歯・口腔・顎顔面に異常を来す疾患・症候群

231. basal cell nevus syndrome: An autosomal dominant syndrome characterized by myriad basal cell nevi with development of basal cell carcinomas in adult life, odontogenic keratocysts, pits in the palms and soles, calcification of the cerebral falx, and bifid ribs.

900 **basal cell nevus syndrome** [béis(ə)l sél ní:vəs síndròum] 名 基底細胞母斑症候群

901 **basal cell** [béis(ə)l sél] 名 基底細胞

902 **dominant** [dámənənt] 形 優性の ↔ recessive (883)

903 **pit** [pít] 名 小窩

904 **palm** [pá:m] 名 手掌

905 **sole** [sóul] 名 足底

906 **cerebral falx** [sərí:br(ə)l fælks] 名 大脳鎌

907 **bifid rib** [báifid ríb] 名 二分肋骨

基底細胞母斑症候群：成人期に基底細胞癌に移行する多数の基底細胞母斑，歯原性角化嚢胞，手掌と足底の小窩，大脳鎌の石灰化，二分肋骨等を特徴とする常染色体優性遺伝による症候群．

---

232. Peutz-Jeghers syndrome: Hamartomatous polyposis of the intestinal tract, associated with melanin spots of the lips, buccal mucosa, hands, and feet.

908 **Peutz-Jeghers syndrome** [pɔ́:ts dʒéigərz síndròum] 名 ポイツ・ジェガース症候群

909 **polyposis** [pɑ̀lipóusəs] 名 ポリープ症

910 **intestinal tract** [intéstən(ə)l trækt] 名 腸管

ポイツ・ジェガース症候群：腸管の過誤腫性ポリープ症で，口唇，頬粘膜，手足のメラニン沈着斑をともなう．

14. 歯・口腔・顎顔面に異常を来す疾患・症候群

233. <u>Gardner syndrome</u>：An autosomal dominant form of polyposis characterized by multiple polyps in the colon together with tumors outside the colon that include osteomas of the skull and mandible, thyroid cancer, epidermoid cysts, fibromas, and desmoid tumors.

911 <u>Gardner syndrome</u>
[gáːrdnər síndròum]
名 ガードナー症候群

912 polyp
[páləp]
名 ポリープ

913 colon
[kóulən]
名 結腸

914 osteoma
[àstióumə]
名 骨腫

915 skull
[skʎl]
名 頭蓋 = cranium (837)

916 thyroid cancer
[θáiərɔ̀id kǽnsər]
名 甲状腺癌

917 desmoid tumor
[dézmɔ̀id t(j)úːmər]
名 デスモイド腫瘍

> **ガードナー症候群**：常染色体優性遺伝によるポリープ症の一形態．結腸内の多発性ポリープおよび結腸外腫瘍（頭蓋・下顎骨腫，甲状腺癌，類表皮嚢胞，線維腫，デスモイド腫瘍等を含む）を特徴とする．

234. <u>von Recklinghausen disease (=neurofibromatosis type 1)</u>：An autosomal dominant disorder characterized by multiple neurofibromas, café-au-lait spots, and osseous lesions.

918 <u>von Recklinghausen disease</u>
[fɑn rékliŋhàuzən dizíːz]
名 フォン・レックリングハウゼン病

919 <u>neurofibromatosis type 1</u>
[n(j)ùəroufàibroumətóusəs táip wʎn]
名 神経線維腫症1型

920 neurofibroma
[n(j)ùəroufaibróumə]
名 神経線維腫

921 café-au-lait spot
[kæféi ou léi spʎt]
名 カフェオレ斑

14. 歯・口腔・顎顔面に異常を来す疾患・症候群

922 **osseous**
[ásiəs]

形 骨の

> フォン・レックリングハウゼン病（＝神経線維腫症1型）：多発性神経線維腫，カフェオレ斑，骨病変等を特徴とする常染色体優性遺伝による疾患．

235. Sturge-Weber syndrome：A congenital disorder characterized by port-wine stains of the face, glaucoma, epilepsy, mental retardation, and leptomeningeal angioma.

923 **Sturge-Weber syndrome**
[stə́ːrdʒ wébər síndròum]

名 スタージ・ウェーバー症候群

924 **port-wine stain**
[pɔ́ːrt wáin stéin]

名 ぶどう酒様血管腫

925 **glaucoma**
[glɔːkóumə]

名 緑内障

926 **epilepsy**
[épəlèpsi]

名 てんかん

927 **mental retardation**
[mént(ə)l rìːtɑːrdéiʃ(ə)n]

名 精神遅滞

928 **leptomeningeal**
[lèptoumənínd ʒiəl]

形 軟膜の

929 **angioma**
[ændʒióumə]

名 血管腫

> スタージ・ウェーバー症候群：顔面のぶどう酒様血管腫，緑内障，てんかん，精神遅滞，軟膜血管腫等を特徴とする先天性疾患．

236. Russell-Silver syndrome：A form of primordial dwarfism characterized by low birth weight, late closure of the anterior fontanel, limb asymmetry, triangular facies, and carp mouth.

930 **Russell-Silver syndrome**
[rʌ́səl sílvər síndròum]

名 ラッセル・シルヴァー症候群

931 **primordial dwarfism**
[praimɔ́ːrdiəl dwɔ́ːrfizm]

名 原発性低身長症

14. 歯・口腔・顎顔面に異常を来す疾患・症候群

932 □ low birth weight
[lóu bə́:rθ wéit]

名 低出生体重

933 □ anterior fontanel
[æntíəriər fὰntənél]

名 大泉門

934 □ facies
[féiʃiì:z]

名 顔貌

935 □ carp mouth
[ká:rp máuθ]

名 鯉口

> **ラッセル・シルヴァー症候群**：低出生体重，大泉門閉鎖遅延，四肢非対称，三角形の顔貌，鯉口等を特徴とする原発性低身長症の一形態．

237. <u>Turner syndrome</u>：A syndrome caused by complete or partial absence of one of the two X chromosomes in females, characterized by short stature, a webbed neck, skeletal abnormalities, and infertility.

936 □ <u>Turner syndrome</u>
[tə́:rnər síndròum]

名 ターナー症候群

937 □ X chromosome
[éks króuməsòum]

名 X 染色体

938 □ chromosome
[króuməsòum]

名 染色体

939 □ short stature
[ʃɔ́:rt stǽtʃər]

名 低身長

940 □ webbed neck
[wébd nék]

名 翼状頸

941 □ infertility
[infərtíləti]

名 不妊

> **ターナー症候群**：女性の 2 本の X 染色体のうちの 1 本が完全に（または一部分のみ）欠損することに起因する症候群．低身長，翼状頸，骨格異常，不妊等を特徴とする．

14. 歯・口腔・顎顔面に異常を来す疾患・症候群

238. Beckwith-Wiedemann syndrome (=EMG syndrome)：A congenital syndrome characterized by exomphalos, macroglossia, and gigantism, often with neonatal hypoglycemia.

942 □ **Beckwith-Wiedemann syndrome**
[békwəθ wíːdəmən síndròum]
名 ベックウィズ・ヴィーデマン症候群

943 □ **EMG syndrome**
[íːèmdʒíː síndròum]
名 EMG 症候群

944 □ **exomphalos**
[eksámfəlùs]
名 臍帯ヘルニア

945 □ **gigantism**
[dʒaigǽntìzm]
名 巨人症

946 □ **hypoglycemia**
[hàipouglaisíːmiə]
名 低血糖

> ベックウィズ・ヴィーデマン症候群(= EMG 症候群)：臍帯ヘルニア，巨舌症，巨人症を特徴とする先天性症候群で，しばしば新生児低血糖をともなう．

239. Pierre Robin syndrome：A congenital syndrome characterized by micrognathia, glossoptosis, and cleft palate.

947 □ **Pierre Robin syndrome**
[pjéər rɔːbán síndròum]
名 ピエール・ロバン症候群

948 □ **glossoptosis**
[glàsouptóusəs]
名 舌根沈下

> ピエール・ロバン症候群：小顎症，舌根沈下，口蓋裂を特徴とする先天性症候群．

240. amelogenesis imperfecta：A hereditary ectodermal disorder in which the enamel is defective in structure or deficient in quantity.

949 □ **amelogenesis imperfecta**
[ǽməloudʒénəsəs ìmpərféktə]
名 エナメル質形成不全症

> エナメル質形成不全症：遺伝性の外胚葉性疾患で，エナメル質の構造的欠陥または量的不足をともなう．

14. 歯・口腔・顎顔面に異常を来す疾患・症候群

241. dentinogenesis imperfecta：A hereditary developmental disorder of the dentin characterized by translucent gray to yellow-brown teeth and marked attrition.

950 **dentinogenesis imperfecta**
[dentì:nədʒénəsəs ìmpərféktə]

名 象牙質形成不全症

象牙質形成不全症：透明度の高い灰色から黄褐色の歯や顕著な咬耗等を特徴とする遺伝性の象牙質発育障害．

---

242. dentin dysplasia：A hereditary disorder of the dentin characterized by short roots, obliteration of the pulp chambers and root canals, and mobility and premature loss of teeth.

951 **dentin dysplasia**
[déntən displéiʒ(i)ə]

名 象牙質異形成症

952 **obliteration**
[əblìtəréiʃ(ə)n]

名 閉塞

953 **pulp chamber**
[pʌ́lp tʃéimbər]

名 髄室

954 **root canal**
[rúːt kənǽl]

名 根管

955 **mobility**
[moubíləti]

名 動揺

象牙質異形成症：短根，髄室・根管の閉塞，歯の動揺・早期脱落等を特徴とする象牙質の遺伝性疾患．

---

243. congenital ectodermal dysplasia：A group of hereditary disorders characterized by abnormal development of the teeth, hair, nails, and sweat glands.

956 **congenital ectodermal dysplasia**
[kəndʒénit(ə)l èktoudə́ːrm(ə)l displéiʒ(i)ə]

名 先天性外胚葉形成不全，先天性外胚葉異形成症

先天性外胚葉形成不全（＝先天性外胚葉異形成症）：歯，毛髪，爪，汗腺等の形成異常を特徴とする遺伝性疾患の一群．

14. 歯・口腔・顎顔面に異常を来す疾患・症候群

244. **incontinentia pigmenti**: A rare genodermatosis characterized by hyperpigmented lesions in linear, zebra stripe, or other bizarre configurations; occasionally accompanied by abnormal development of the eyes, teeth, nails, skeleton, and heart.

957 **incontinentia pigmenti** [inkùntənénʃ(i)ə pigméntai]
名 色素失調症

958 **genodermatosis** [dʒì:noudə̀:rmətóusəs]
名 遺伝性皮膚疾患

959 **hyperpigmented** [hàipərpígməntid]
形 色素沈着過剰の → hyperpigmentation (648)

> **色素失調症**：線状，シマウマ模様，その他の奇異な形状の色素沈着過剰性の病変を特徴とするまれな遺伝性皮膚疾患．ときに目，歯，爪，骨格，心臓等の形成異常をともなう．

245. **hypophosphatasia**: A rare congenital disorder associated with a low level of serum alkaline phosphatase, hyperphosphaturia, hypercalcemia, skeletal abnormalities, pathologic fractures, craniostenosis, and premature loss of teeth.

960 **hypophosphatasia** [hàipoufàsfətéiʒ(i)ə]
名 低フォスファターゼ症

961 **serum** [síərəm]
名 血清，漿液

962 **alkaline phosphatase** [ǽlkəlàin fásfətèis]
名 アルカリフォスファターゼ

963 **hyperphosphaturia** [hàipərfùsfət(j)úəriə]
名 高リン酸塩尿症

964 **hypercalcemia** [hàipərkælsí:miə]
名 高カルシウム血症

965 **pathologic fracture** [pæ̀θəládʒik frǽktʃər]
名 病的骨折

966 **craniostenosis** [krèinioustənóusəs]
名 狭頭症

> **低フォスファターゼ症**：血清アルカリフォスファターゼ低値，高リン酸塩尿症，高カルシウム血症，骨格異常，病的骨折，狭頭症，歯の早期脱落等をともなうまれな先天性疾患．

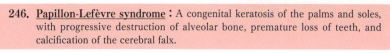

14. 歯・口腔・顎顔面に異常を来す疾患・症候群

246. **Papillon-Lefèvre syndrome**：A congenital keratosis of the palms and soles, with progressive destruction of alveolar bone, premature loss of teeth, and calcification of the cerebral falx.

967 □ **Papillon-Lefèvre syndrome**
[pɑ̀ːpijɔ́ːŋ ləfévrə síndròum]
名 パピヨン・ルフェーヴル症候群

968 □ keratosis
[kèrətóusəs]
名 角化症

> パピヨン・ルフェーヴル症候群：手掌と足底の先天性角化症で，歯槽骨の進行性破壊，歯の早期脱落，大脳鎌の石灰化等をともなう．

247. **Down syndrome (=trisomy 21 syndrome)**：A syndrome due to the presence of an extra chromosome 21, characterized by mental retardation, short stature, microcephaly, flat face, and decreased muscle tone.

969 □ **Down syndrome**
[dáun síndròum]
名 ダウン症候群

970 □ trisomy 21 syndrome
[tráisòumi twéntiwʌ́n síndròum]
名 21 トリソミー症候群

971 □ microcephaly
[màikrouséfəli]
名 小頭症

972 □ muscle tone
[mʌ́s(ə)l tóun]
名 筋緊張

> ダウン症候群(=21 トリソミー症候群)：21 番染色体が1本余分に存在することに起因する症候群．精神遅滞，低身長，小頭症，扁平な顔，筋緊張低下等を特徴とする．

248. **Klinefelter syndrome**：A syndrome due to the presence of one or more extra X chromosomes in males, characterized by small testes, azoospermia, gynecomastia, and long limbs.

973 □ **Klinefelter syndrome**
[kláinfèltər síndròum]
名 クラインフェルター症候群

974 □ testes
[téstìːz]
名 精巣（複；単 testis [téstəs]）

975 □ azoospermia
[eizòuəspə́ːrmiə]
名 無精子症

976 □ gynecomastia
[gàinikoumǽstiə]
名 女性化乳房

14. 歯・口腔・顎顔面に異常を来す疾患・症候群

> **クラインフェルター症候群**：男性のX染色体が1本以上余分に存在することに起因する症候群．小さい精巣，無精子症，女性化乳房，長い四肢等を特徴とする．

249. trisomy 18 syndrome (=Edwards syndrome)：A syndrome due to the presence of an extra chromosome 18, characterized by mental retardation, microcephaly, low-set ears, micrognathia, prominent occiput, and abnormal flexion of fingers.

977 trisomy 18 syndrome [tráisòumi èití:n síndròum] — 名 18トリソミー症候群

978 Edwards syndrome [édwərdz síndròum] — 名 エドワーズ症候群

979 occiput [ɑ́ksəpət] — 名 後頭部

980 flexion [flékʃ(ə)n] — 名 屈曲

> **18トリソミー症候群（＝エドワーズ症候群）**：18番染色体が1本余分に存在することに起因する症候群．精神遅滞，小頭症，耳介低位，小顎症，後頭部の突出，手指の屈曲異常等を特徴とする．

250. cri du chat syndrome：A syndrome due to deletion of the short arm of chromosome 5, characterized by microcephaly, hypertelorism, downwardly slanting palpebral fissures, micrognathia, strabismus, mental retardation, and a high-pitched catlike cry.

981 cri du chat syndrome [krì: du ʃá: síndròum] — 名 猫鳴き症候群

982 deletion [dilí:ʃ(ə)n] — 名 欠失

983 short arm [ʃɔ́:rt á:rm] — 名 短腕

984 strabismus [strəbízməs] — 名 斜視

> **猫鳴き症候群**：5番染色体の短腕の欠失に起因する症候群．小頭症，両眼隔離，眼瞼裂の下方傾斜，小顎症，斜視，精神遅滞，高音のネコ様の泣き声等を特徴とする．

関連語

985 □ microdontia
[màikroudánʃiə]
名 小歯症

986 □ macrodontia
[mæ̀krondánʃiə]
名 巨歯症

987 □ early eruption
[ə́:rli irʌ́pʃ(ə)n]
名 早期萌出 ↔ delayed eruption (81)

988 □ tartar
[tá:rtər]
名 歯石 = dental calculus (198)

989 □ heredity
[hərédəti]
名 遺伝

990 □ mental
[mént(ə)l]
形 オトガイの

991 □ tonsillitis
[tànsəláitəs]
名 扁桃炎

992 □ cuspid
[kʌ́spəd]
名 尖頭歯 = canine (348)

993 □ aneurysm
[ǽnjərìzm]
名 動脈瘤

994 □ ameloblast
[ǽməloublæ̀st]
名 エナメル芽細胞

995 □ hamartoma
[hæ̀mà:rtóumə]
名 過誤腫

996 □ antibody
[ǽntibàdi]
名 抗体

997 □ epidermis
[èpədə́:rməs]
名 表皮

998 □ gangrene
[gǽŋgri:n]
名 壊疽

999 □ sympathetic
[sìmpəθétik]
形 交感神経の ↔ parasympathetic (781)

1000 □ palpebra
[pǽlpəbrə]
名 眼瞼 = eyelid (854)

英語索引

A

- aberrant salivary gland 758
- abfraction 130
- abrasion 124
- abrasion 696
- abscess 188
- accessory salivary gland 757
- achondroplasia 863
- acid 118
- acinar 485
- acinar cell 503
- acinic cell carcinoma 500
- acquired 240
- acrocephalosyndactyly 862
- *Actinomyces* 306
- actinomycosis 305
- acute 181
- Addison's disease 644
- adenoid cystic carcinoma 490
- adenoma 463
- adenomatoid odontogenic tumor 423
- adrenocortical 645
- ageusia 804
- AIDS 636
- alar cartilage 889
- alkaline phosphatase 962
- allergen 691
- allergy 620
- alveolar 200
- alveolar bone 201
- alveolar cleft 214
- alveolar mucosa 340
- alveolar osteitis 702
- alveolar process 215
- alveolus 140
- ameloblast 994
- ameloblastic 432
- ameloblastic fibroma 431
- ameloblastic fibrosarcoma 459
- ameloblastoma 419
- amelogenesis imperfecta 949
- amyloid 429
- anemia 595
- aneurysm 993
- aneurysmal 374
- aneurysmal bone cyst 373
- angina 288
- angioedema 601
- angioma 929
- angle of mouth 618
- angular cheilitis 651
- angular stomatitis 650
- ankyloglossia 278
- ankylosis 756
- anodontia 8
- anorexia 649
- anterior 89
- anterior fontanel 933
- anterior lingual gland 396
- anterior teeth 90
- antibody 996
- antipsychotic agent 828
- anus 579
- aortic dissection 897
- Apert syndrome 861
- aperture 242
- apex 395
- aphtha 698
- aphthous 609
- apical 157
- apical periodontitis 162
- appendage 399
- arachnodactyly 895
- arthralgia 585
- arthritis 591
- articular 724
- articular cartilage 725
- articular chondrocalcinosis 748
- asymptomatic 382
- atopic dermatitis 656
- atrophic 599
- atrophic glossitis 660
- atrophy 176
- attached gingiva 347
- attrition 122
- auricle 855
- auriculotemporal nerve 782
- autoantibody 565
- autoimmune 563
- autoimmune disease 564
- autosomal 882
- azoospermia 975

B

- bacteria 711
- bacterial 654
- bald tongue 662
- basal cell 901
- basal cell nevus syndrome 900
- Beckwith-Wiedemann syndrome 942
- Bednar's aphthae 697
- Behçet disease 611
- Bell's palsy 818
- benign 370
- benign lymphoepithelial lesion 473
- bifid rib 907
- bifid tongue 886
- bifurcation 48
- bilateral 247
- bimaxillary protrusion 106
- bisphosphonate 714
- bisphosphonate-related osteonecrosis of the jaw (BRONJ) 713
- black hairy tongue 669
- Blandin-Nuhn cyst 394
- bleeding 171
- blood vessel 158
- bone density 841
- bone marrow 709
- bone resorption 842
- brachydactyly 891
- brainstem 812
- branchial arch 872
- branchial cleft 412

- ☐ branchial cyst 409
- ☐ bruxism 132
- ☐ buccal 25
- ☐ buccal mucosa 489
- ☐ bullae 568
- ☐ bullous 588
- ☐ burning pain 739

C

- ☐ café-au-lait spot 921
- ☐ calcification 327
- ☐ calcified 145
- ☐ calcifying cystic odontogenic tumor 441
- ☐ calcifying epithelial odontogenic tumor 426
- ☐ calcium pyrophosphate 750
- ☐ calculi 785
- ☐ cancer 487
- ☐ *Candida albicans* 630
- ☐ candidiasis 629
- ☐ canine 348
- ☐ capillary 605
- ☐ Carabelli's tubercle 18
- ☐ carbohydrate 121
- ☐ carcinoma 457
- ☐ cardiovascular 896
- ☐ carp mouth 935
- ☐ cartilage 726
- ☐ cartilaginous 755
- ☐ caseous 319
- ☐ caseous necrosis 320
- ☐ cellulitis 283
- ☐ cementoblastoma 453
- ☐ cementoenamel junction 47
- ☐ cementum 14
- ☐ central incisor 6
- ☐ centric occlusion 94
- ☐ cerebral falx 906
- ☐ cerebrum 811
- ☐ cervical 40
- ☐ cervical margin 41
- ☐ cheilitis 679
- ☐ cherubism 529
- ☐ chewing 794
- ☐ chill 707
- ☐ chondrocalcinosis 749
- ☐ chondromatosis 754
- ☐ chromosome 938
- ☐ chronic 154
- ☐ chronic periodontitis 196
- ☐ chronic pulpitis 155
- ☐ chronic sclerosing submandibular sialadenitis 480
- ☐ circumvallate papillae 675
- ☐ clavicle 835
- ☐ cleft lip 208
- ☐ cleft palate 216
- ☐ cleft tongue 253
- ☐ cleidocranial dysostosis 833
- ☐ cleidocranial dysplasia 832
- ☐ clinodactyly 892
- ☐ collagen 845
- ☐ coloboma 853
- ☐ colon 913
- ☐ complex odontoma 440
- ☐ complex regional pain syndrome（CRPS）801
- ☐ complication 416
- ☐ compound 51
- ☐ compound odontoma 439
- ☐ concrescent teeth 13
- ☐ congenital 9
- ☐ congenital ectodermal dysplasia 956
- ☐ congenital epulis 512
- ☐ congenital tooth 79
- ☐ congenital velopharyngeal insufficiency 231
- ☐ congestion 150
- ☐ conical tooth 38
- ☐ connective tissue 297
- ☐ constitutional symptom 712
- ☐ contact cheilitis 689
- ☐ contagious 772
- ☐ contraction 823
- ☐ coronal 32
- ☐ Costen syndrome 736
- ☐ coxsackievirus 554
- ☐ cranial 107
- ☐ cranial base 108
- ☐ cranial nerve 824
- ☐ craniofacial dysostosis 857
- ☐ craniostenosis 966
- ☐ craniosynostosis 858
- ☐ cranium 837
- ☐ cri du chat syndrome 981
- ☐ crossbite 85
- ☐ Crouzon syndrome 856
- ☐ crowding 101
- ☐ crown 16
- ☐ crystal 747
- ☐ cusp 22
- ☐ cuspid 992
- ☐ cutaneous 311
- ☐ cyclosporine 273
- ☐ cyst 322
- ☐ cystic 324
- ☐ cytoplasm 469

D

- ☐ deciduous tooth 63
- ☐ deficiency 653
- ☐ deformity 741
- ☐ degeneration 325
- ☐ delayed eruption 81
- ☐ deletion 982
- ☐ dens in dente 28
- ☐ dental arch 72
- ☐ dental calculus 198
- ☐ dental caries 111
- ☐ dental fistula 191
- ☐ dental floss 127
- ☐ dental follicle 446
- ☐ dental lamina 262
- ☐ dental papilla 445
- ☐ dental plaque 168
- ☐ dental pulp 148
- ☐ denticle 143
- ☐ dentigerous cyst 335
- ☐ dentin 11
- ☐ dentin dysplasia 951
- ☐ dentin hypersensitivity 141
- ☐ dentinogenesis imperfecta 950
- ☐ denture 514
- ☐ denture fibroma 513
- ☐ deposit 430
- ☐ deposition 639

☐ dermatitis	657
☐ dermis	685
☐ dermoid cyst	397
☐ desmoid tumor	917
☐ desquamation	177
☐ desquamative gingivitis	172
☐ detachment	589
☐ developmental disorder	55
☐ deviation	87
☐ differentiation	504
☐ diffuse	269
☐ dilatation	603
☐ discoid lupus erythematosus (DLE)	596
☐ discoloration	670
☐ dissolution	114
☐ dominant	902
☐ dorsal	668
☐ dorsum	671
☐ double lip	239
☐ Down syndrome	969
☐ draining sinus	307
☐ drifting	99
☐ dry mouth	761
☐ duct	390
☐ dwarfism	865
☐ dysfunction	526
☐ dysgeusia	829
☐ dyskinesia	827
☐ dysostosis	834
☐ dysphagia	557
☐ dysplasia	520

E

☐ ear canal	817
☐ early eruption	987
☐ ectodermal	398
☐ ectopia lentis	899
☐ ectopic	256
☐ edema	249
☐ edematous	575
☐ edge-to-edge occlusion	96
☐ Edwards syndrome	978
☐ effusion	735
☐ embryogenesis	414
☐ embryonic	213

☐ EMG syndrome	943
☐ enamel	33
☐ enamel drop	44
☐ enamel epithelium	338
☐ enamel hypoplasia	54
☐ enamel organ	326
☐ enamel pearl	45
☐ endocrine	251
☐ enterovirus	559
☐ enzymatic	119
☐ eosinophilic	471
☐ epibulbar	876
☐ epidemic	771
☐ epidemic parotitis	769
☐ epidermal	587
☐ epidermis	997
☐ epidermoid cell	498
☐ epidermoid cyst	403
☐ epidermolysis bullosa	573
☐ epilepsy	926
☐ epimyoepithelial island	478
☐ epithelial	258
☐ epithelial pearls	257
☐ epithelioid cell	684
☐ epithelium	334
☐ epulis	505
☐ epulis granulomatosa	507
☐ erosion	128
☐ erosion	537
☐ erosive	627
☐ erupt	74
☐ erupted	3
☐ eruption	82
☐ eruption	550
☐ eruption cyst	339
☐ erythema	174
☐ erythema multiforme	574
☐ erythema nodosum	614
☐ erythematous	666
☐ erythroplakia	634
☐ etiology	474
☐ exomphalos	944
☐ exomphthalmos	860
☐ external resorption	160
☐ extraction	300
☐ exudate	610
☐ eyelid	854

F

☐ facial asymmetry	719
☐ facial cleft	221
☐ facial muscles	807
☐ facial nerve	688
☐ facial paralysis	805
☐ facial spasm	820
☐ facies	934
☐ fauces	555
☐ fever	58
☐ fibroblastic	444
☐ fibroma	433
☐ fibromatosis	264
☐ fibromatous epulis	508
☐ fibro-osseous	521
☐ fibrosarcoma	460
☐ fibrous	266
☐ fibrous connective tissue	447
☐ filiform papillae	664
☐ first and second branchial arch syndrome	871
☐ first molar	70
☐ fissure	209
☐ fissured tongue	667
☐ fistula	192
☐ flange	515
☐ flexion	980
☐ floor of mouth	293
☐ fluorine	50
☐ fluorosis	49
☐ flushing	779
☐ follicular	337
☐ follicular dental cyst	336
☐ Fordyce spots	676
☐ Fournier teeth	68
☐ fracture	138
☐ fragility	846
☐ free gingiva	346
☐ frenulum	280
☐ Frey syndrome	778
☐ frontal bossing	866
☐ fused teeth	10

G

- ganglion 815
- gangrene 998
- gangrenous 617
- gangrenous stomatitis 615
- Gardner syndrome 911
- geminated tooth 15
- generalized 840
- geniculate ganglion 814
- genital 612
- genitals 580
- genodermatosis 958
- genu varum 870
- geographic tongue 672
- ghost cell 442
- giant cell 380
- giant cell epulis 510
- gigantism 945
- gingiva 167
- gingival 136
- gingival abscess 187
- gingival cyst 345
- gingival fibromatosis 263
- gingival hyperplasia 268
- gingival margin 137
- gingival recession 206
- gingivitis 166
- gingivostomatitis 535
- gland 385
- glandular 351
- glandular odontogenic cyst 350
- glandular tissue 496
- glaucoma 925
- glossitis 661
- glossodynia 803
- glossopharyngeal nerve 797
- glossopharyngeal neuralgia 796
- glossoptosis 948
- Goldenhar syndrome 875
- gout 742
- granular 470
- granuloma 318
- granulomatous cheilitis 682
- growth 506
- gynecomastia 976

H

- hair follicle 402
- hairy leukoplakia 635
- halitosis 182
- hamartoma 995
- hamartomatous 438
- hand-foot-and-mouth disease 558
- hard palate 228
- hard tissue 436
- headache 584
- hearing loss 737
- hemangioma 237
- hemorrhage 371
- hereditary 270
- heredity 989
- herpangina 553
- herpes 539
- herpes labialis 542
- herpes simplex virus 540
- herpes zoster 545
- herpetic 534
- herpetic gingivostomatitis 533
- high-arched palate 275
- histologic 491
- Hunter's glossitis 663
- Hutchinson teeth 66
- hypercalcemia 964
- hyperemia 147
- hyperkeratosis 633
- hyperphosphaturia 963
- hyperpigmentation 648
- hyperpigmented 959
- hyperplasia 267
- hypersensitivity 142
- hypertelorism 859
- hypertrophy 245
- hyperuricemia 745
- hypoglycemia 946
- hypophosphatasia 960
- hypoplasia 52
- hypoplastic 888
- hyposecretion 767
- hypotension 647
- hypothyroidism 236

I

- idiopathic 673
- impacted tooth 73
- incisal edge 42
- incisive canal 357
- incisor 7
- incontinentia pigmenti 957
- indentation 383
- infant 695
- infection 292
- inferior 359
- infertility 941
- infiltration 477
- inflammation 62
- inflammatory 364
- injury 205
- inorganic 115
- insufficiency 646
- intercellular adhesion molecule 566
- interdental papillae 184
- intermediate cell 499
- internal resorption 161
- intestinal tract 910
- intraosseous 427
- invaginate 34
- invasive 450
- involuntary 822
- iron deficiency anemia 659
- irritant 690

J

- jaw 84
- joint 722
- joint laxity 848

K

- keratinized 404
- keratinized stratified squamous epithelium 405
- keratoconjunctivitis 776
- keratoconjunctivitis sicca 777
- keratocyst 329

- ☐ keratocystic odontogenic tumor — 421
- ☐ keratosis — 968
- ☐ Klinefelter syndrome — 973
- ☐ Koplik spots — 560
- ☐ Küttner's tumor — 481

L

- ☐ labial — 86
- ☐ labial mucosa — 680
- ☐ lacrimal gland — 475
- ☐ Langerhans cell histiocytosis — 530
- ☐ latent — 547
- ☐ lateral — 30
- ☐ lateral cervical cyst — 410
- ☐ lateral incisor — 31
- ☐ lateral periodontal cyst — 341
- ☐ leptomeningeal — 928
- ☐ lesion — 135
- ☐ leukoplakia — 631
- ☐ lichen — 622
- ☐ lichen planus — 623
- ☐ ligament — 203
- ☐ limb — 864
- ☐ line — 330
- ☐ lingual — 20
- ☐ lingual frenulum — 279
- ☐ lingual thyroid — 254
- ☐ lingual tonsil — 678
- ☐ lingual tonsil hypertrophy — 677
- ☐ lip sucking habit — 235
- ☐ lipodermoid — 877
- ☐ lobulated tongue — 885
- ☐ lobule — 789
- ☐ localized — 113
- ☐ long bone — 377
- ☐ lordosis — 869
- ☐ low birth weight — 932
- ☐ low-grade — 501
- ☐ Ludwig's angina — 287
- ☐ lumbar — 868
- ☐ lupus — 310
- ☐ lupus vulgaris — 309
- ☐ luxation — 139
- ☐ lymph node — 317
- ☐ lymphadenitis — 316
- ☐ lymphangioma — 238
- ☐ lymphocyte — 476
- ☐ lymphoepithelial cyst — 411
- ☐ lymphoid tissue — 467

M

- ☐ macrocheilia — 234
- ☐ macrodont — 37
- ☐ macrodontia — 986
- ☐ macroglossia — 248
- ☐ macule — 598
- ☐ malaise — 583
- ☐ malformation — 29
- ☐ malignant — 458
- ☐ malnutrition — 57
- ☐ malocclusion — 83
- ☐ malposed — 887
- ☐ mammary gland — 493
- ☐ mandible — 93
- ☐ mandibular — 27
- ☐ mandibular condylar hyperplasia — 717
- ☐ mandibular condyle — 718
- ☐ mandibular protrusion — 105
- ☐ mandibular retrusion — 109
- ☐ mandibular torus — 518
- ☐ mandibulofacial dysostosis — 850
- ☐ marble bone disease — 839
- ☐ Marfan syndrome — 893
- ☐ marginal gingiva — 186
- ☐ marginal periodontitis — 304
- ☐ masseter muscle — 244
- ☐ masseter muscle hypertrophy — 243
- ☐ matrix — 56
- ☐ maxilla — 91
- ☐ maxillary — 5
- ☐ maxillary process — 212
- ☐ maxillary protrusion — 103
- ☐ maxillary sinus — 303
- ☐ McCune-Albright syndrome — 522
- ☐ measles — 561
- ☐ medial — 210
- ☐ median — 222
- ☐ median cervical cyst — 407
- ☐ median facial cleft — 223
- ☐ median rhomboid glossitis — 674
- ☐ melanin — 640
- ☐ melanism — 638
- ☐ Melkersson-Rosenthal syndrome — 686
- ☐ membrane — 343
- ☐ mental — 990
- ☐ mental retardation — 927
- ☐ mesenchymal — 434
- ☐ mesiobuccal — 26
- ☐ mesiodens — 2
- ☐ mesiolingual — 21
- ☐ metabolic — 271
- ☐ metabolism — 744
- ☐ metaplasia — 788
- ☐ microcephaly — 971
- ☐ microdont — 36
- ☐ microdontia — 985
- ☐ microglossia — 252
- ☐ micrognathia — 879
- ☐ microorganism — 120
- ☐ microstomia — 241
- ☐ midpalatal — 700
- ☐ migrate — 874
- ☐ Mikulicz disease — 774
- ☐ mitochondria — 472
- ☐ mitral valve prolapse — 898
- ☐ mobility — 955
- ☐ molar — 23
- ☐ molecule — 567
- ☐ Moon teeth — 69
- ☐ motor nucleus — 825
- ☐ mottled tooth — 53
- ☐ mucocele — 387
- ☐ mucocutaneous — 571
- ☐ mucoepidermoid carcinoma — 495
- ☐ mucosa — 194
- ☐ mucosal — 175
- ☐ mucous — 388
- ☐ mucous cell — 497
- ☐ mucous cyst — 386

mucous gland	391
mucous membrane	569
mucus	492
multifocal	532
multilocular	353
multinucleated	379
multiple	259
multisystemic	894
mumps	770
muscle	229
muscle tone	972
myxoid	451
myxoma	449

N

nasal ala	360
nasal bridge	890
nasal process	211
nasoalveolar cyst	358
nasolacrimal duct	361
nasopalatine duct	356
nasopalatine duct cyst	355
neck of tooth	207
necrosis	153
necrotizing	179
necrotizing sialometaplasia	786
necrotizing ulcerative gingivitis	178
neonatal	80
neonate	260
neoplasm	488
nerve	552
neural crest	873
neuralgia	791
neuralgic	549
neurofibroma	920
neurofibromatosis type 1	919
neuropathic	802
nevus	642
nevus pigmentosus	641
nicotine stomatitis	637
nifedipine	274
nodular	313
nodule	46
noma	616

noncaseating	683
noninflammatory	265
nonvital tooth	366
nostril	578
notched	67
nucleus	808
nutritional	652

O

oblique facial cleft	225
obliteration	952
occiput	979
occlusal	77
occlusal force	131
occlusal plane	78
occlusal surface	123
occlusal trauma	204
occlusal vertical dimension	98
occlusion	95,156
odontogenesis	65
odontogenic	295
odontogenic cyst	323
odontogenic fibroma	443
odontogenic keratocyst	328
odontogenic maxillary sinusitis	301
odontogenic myxoma	448
odontogenic peritonsillitis	294
odontoma	437
oncocytoma	468
open bite	88
opposing teeth	92
oral cancer	486
oral candidiasis	628
oral cavity	219
oral dyskinesia	826
oral-facial-digital syndrome	881
oral lichen planus	621
oral mucosa	193
organic	116
organic acid	117
orthokeratinized	331
osseous	922

osseous dysplasia	519
ossification	836
ossifying epulis	509
osteitis	703
osteoarthritis	723
osteochondroma	752
osteoclast	843
osteogenesis imperfecta	844
osteolytic	376
osteoma	914
osteomyelitis	708
osteonecrosis	715
osteopetrosis	838
osteophyte	727
overbite	100
overclosure	97

P

pain	173
palatal torus	516
palate	217
palatine process	220
palm	904
palpebra	1000
palpebral	851
palpebral fissure	852
palsy	819
papilla	185
papillary	466
Papillon-Lefèvre syndrome	967
papular	625
papule	576
paradental cyst	368
parakeratinized	422
paralysis	687
paramyxovirus	773
parasympathetic	781
parenchyma	479
paresis	806
parotid gland	413
paroxysmal	792
pathologic fracture	965
pathological	784
peg tooth	39
pemphigoid	570

- pemphigus 562
- periapical 365
- periarticular 732
- pericarditis 593
- pericoronitis 281
- periductal 483
- periodontal 164
- periodontal ligament 202
- periodontal membrane 342
- periodontal pocket 199
- periodontitis 163
- periodontium 197
- perioral 544
- periosteum 705
- periostitis 704
- peripheral 809
- peritonsillitis 296
- permanent tooth 61
- permeability 604
- Peutz-Jeghers syndrome 908
- pharynx 798
- phenytoin 272
- Pierre Robin syndrome 947
- pigmentation 525
- pigmented 643
- pit 903
- plaque 626
- pleomorphic adenoma 462
- pleuritis 592
- Plummer-Vinson syndrome 658
- polyostotic fibrous dysplasia 524
- polyp 912
- polyposis 909
- port-wine stain 924
- posterior 110
- postoperative maxillary cyst 415
- preauricular 878
- precancerous 632
- precocious puberty 527
- pregnancy epulis 511
- premolar 349
- primary 455
- primary intraosseous squamous cell carcinoma 454
- primordial cyst 321
- primordial dwarfism 931
- proliferation 428
- protostylid 24
- pruritic 572
- puberty 528
- pulp cavity 35
- pulp chamber 953
- pulp hyperemia 146
- pulp necrosis 152
- pulp stone 144
- pulpitis 151
- purine 743
- purulent 734
- pus 189
- pyogenic 710

Q

- Quincke's edema 602

R

- radical surgery 417
- radicular 363
- radicular cyst 362
- radiograph 354
- radiolucency 425
- radiolucent 461
- Ramsay Hunt syndrome 813
- ramus 420
- ranula 392
- raphe 701
- reactivation 546
- recessive 883
- recurrent 608
- recurrent aphthous stomatitis 607
- redness 169
- remnant 261
- renal 594
- residual cyst 367
- respiratory tract 494
- retention cyst 389
- reticular 624
- rheumatoid arthritis 740
- Riga-Fede disease 692
- root 17
- root apex 165
- root canal 954
- root of tongue 799
- root resorption 159
- Russell-Silver syndrome 930

S

- saddle nose 867
- saliva 763
- salivary fistula 759
- salivary gland 464
- scalp 597
- scar 600
- sclera 847
- sclerosis 484
- sebaceous gland 400
- secretion 762
- sense of taste 830
- sensitivity 831
- sensory nerve 551
- septicemia 308
- serous 502
- serum 961
- short arm 983
- short stature 939
- sialadenitis 482,765
- sialoangiitis 768
- sialolith 766
- sialolithiasis 783
- sialometaplasia 787
- sialorrhea 764
- side effect 716
- simple bone cyst 369
- sinusitis 302
- Sjögren syndrome 775
- skeletal 276
- skeletal system 277
- skeleton 104
- skin 284
- skull 915
- slough 183
- sodium urate 746
- soft palate 230
- soft tissue 190
- sole 905
- solitary 375

- ☐ sore throat — 556
- ☐ spasm — 821
- ☐ squamous cell — 456
- ☐ squamous epithelium — 333
- ☐ static bone cavity — 381
- ☐ Stevens-Johnson syndrome — 577
- ☐ stiffness — 733
- ☐ stomach acid — 129
- ☐ stomatitis medicamentosa — 619
- ☐ strabismus — 984
- ☐ stratified squamous epithelium — 332
- ☐ stroma — 452
- ☐ Sturge-Weber syndrome — 923
- ☐ subcutaneous — 285
- ☐ subcutaneous tissue — 286
- ☐ sublingual — 290
- ☐ sublingual gland — 393
- ☐ submandibular gland — 384
- ☐ submaxillary — 289
- ☐ submental — 291
- ☐ submerged tooth — 76
- ☐ submucous — 227
- ☐ submucous cleft palate — 226
- ☐ superior — 218
- ☐ superior pharyngeal constrictor muscle — 233
- ☐ supernumerary tooth — 1
- ☐ suppurative — 195
- ☐ suppurative arthritis — 731
- ☐ supranuclear — 810
- ☐ surgery — 418
- ☐ swallowing — 800
- ☐ sweat gland — 401
- ☐ sweating — 780
- ☐ swelling — 170
- ☐ sympathetic — 999
- ☐ symptom — 582
- ☐ syndrome — 523
- ☐ synovial — 728
- ☐ synovial chondromatosis — 753
- ☐ synovial fluid — 751
- ☐ synovial membrane — 729
- ☐ syphilis — 59
- ☐ systemic — 581
- ☐ systemic lupus erythematosus (SLE) — 590

T

- ☐ tartar — 988
- ☐ taurodont — 43
- ☐ teethe — 694
- ☐ temporomandibular joint — 721
- ☐ temporomandibular joint disorder — 720
- ☐ tenderness — 706
- ☐ testes — 974
- ☐ third molar — 282
- ☐ thyroglossal duct — 408
- ☐ thyroglossal duct cyst — 406
- ☐ thyroid — 255
- ☐ thyroid cancer — 916
- ☐ tinnitus — 738
- ☐ tissue — 75
- ☐ tonsil — 298
- ☐ tonsillitis — 991
- ☐ tooth bud — 435
- ☐ tooth decay — 112
- ☐ tooth germ — 12
- ☐ toothbrush — 125
- ☐ toothpaste — 133
- ☐ toothpick — 126
- ☐ torsiversion — 102
- ☐ torus — 517
- ☐ toxic epidermal necrolysis (TEN) — 586
- ☐ transverse facial cleft — 224
- ☐ transversion — 71
- ☐ trauma — 64
- ☐ traumatic — 699
- ☐ traumatic arthritis — 730
- ☐ Treacher Collins syndrome — 849
- ☐ trigeminal nerve — 793
- ☐ trigeminal neuralgia — 790
- ☐ trigger point — 795
- ☐ trisomy 18 syndrome — 977
- ☐ trisomy 21 syndrome — 970
- ☐ tubercle — 19
- ☐ tuberculosis — 312
- ☐ tuberculous — 315
- ☐ tuberculous cervical lymphadenitis — 314
- ☐ tumor — 250
- ☐ Turner syndrome — 936
- ☐ Turner tooth — 60

U

- ☐ ulcer — 538
- ☐ ulceration — 693
- ☐ ulcerative — 180
- ☐ unerupted — 4
- ☐ unifocal — 531
- ☐ unilateral — 246
- ☐ unilocular — 352
- ☐ uveitis — 613

V

- ☐ varicella-zoster virus — 548
- ☐ vascular — 149
- ☐ velopharyngeal — 232
- ☐ venous — 372
- ☐ vermilion border — 681
- ☐ vertebra — 378
- ☐ vertebral — 880
- ☐ vertigo — 816
- ☐ vesicle — 543
- ☐ vesicular — 536
- ☐ viral — 655
- ☐ virus — 541
- ☐ vital tooth — 344
- ☐ vitamin — 665
- ☐ von Recklinghausen disease — 918

W

- ☐ Warthin tumor — 465
- ☐ webbed neck — 940
- ☐ wedge-shaped defect — 134
- ☐ well-circumscribed — 424
- ☐ wheal — 606
- ☐ wisdom tooth — 299

X

- X chromosome　937
- xerostomia　760
- X-linked　884

日本語索引

あ

- 悪性の　458
- アジソン病　644
- 圧痛　706
- アトピー性皮膚炎　656
- アフタ　698
- アフタ(性)の　609
- アブフラクション　130
- アペール症候群　861
- アミロイド　429
- アルカリフォスファターゼ　962
- アレルギー　620
- アレルゲン　691
- アンギナ　288
- 鞍鼻　867

い

- EMG症候群　943
- 異形成(症)　520
- 異骨症　834
- 胃酸　129
- 遺残組織　261
- 萎縮　176
- 萎縮(性)の　599
- 萎縮性舌炎　660
- 異所性の　256
- 位置異常の　887
- 遺伝　989
- 遺伝性の　270
- 遺伝性皮膚疾患　958
- 移動　99
- 咽頭　798

- 咽頭痛　556

う

- ウイルス　541
- ウイルス(性)の　655
- ウォーシン腫瘍　465
- う蝕　111,112
- うっ血　150
- 運動核　825

え

- 永久歯　61
- エイズ　636
- 栄養の　652
- 栄養不良　57
- 壊死　153
- 壊死性潰瘍性歯肉炎　178
- 壊死性唾液腺化生　786
- 壊死性の　179
- 壊疽　998
- 壊疽(性)の　617
- 壊疽性口内炎　615
- エックス線写真　354
- X染色体　937
- エックス線透過性の　461
- エックス線透過像　425
- X連鎖の　884
- エドワーズ症候群　978
- エナメル芽細胞　994
- エナメル芽細胞の　432
- エナメル器　326
- エナメル質　33

- エナメル質形成不全症　949
- エナメル質減形成(症)　54
- エナメル上皮　338
- エナメル上皮腫　419
- エナメル上皮線維腫　431
- エナメル上皮線維肉腫　459
- エナメル真珠　45
- エナメル滴　44
- エプーリス　505
- 嚥下　800
- 嚥下困難　557
- 炎症　62
- 炎症性の　364
- 円錐歯　38
- エンテロウイルス　559
- 円板状エリテマトーデス　596

お

- 横顔(面)裂　224
- 悪寒　707
- おたふくかぜ　770
- オトガイ下の　291
- オトガイの　990
- オンコサイトーマ　468

か

- ガードナー症候群　911
- 開咬症　88
- 開口部　242
- 外耳道　817
- 外傷　64
- 外傷(性)の　699

□外傷性関節炎	730	□ガマ腫	392	□基底細胞母斑症候群	900
□外側の	30	□カラベリー結節	18	□気道	494
□外胚葉の	398	□顆粒状の	470	□機能障害，機能不全	526
□外部吸収	160	□癌	457,487	□機能低下	646
□潰瘍	538	□陥凹	383	□丘疹	576
□潰瘍(性)の	180	□感覚神経	551	□丘疹(性)の	625
□潰瘍化	693	□眼球上の	876	□吸唇癖	235
□過蓋咬合	100	□眼球突出	860	□急性の	181
□下顎(骨)	93	□眼瞼	854,1000	□キュットナー腫瘍	481
□下顎(骨)の	27	□眼瞼の	851	□境界明瞭な	424
□下顎顔面異骨症	850	□眼瞼裂	852	□頬側の	25
□下顎後退症	109	□含歯性嚢胞	335	□狭頭症	966
□下顎枝	420	□カンジダ・アルビカンス	630	□頬粘膜	489
□下顎前突症	105	□カンジダ症	629	□強膜	847
□下顎頭,顆頭	718	□感受性	831	□胸膜炎	592
□下顎頭過形成	717	□乾性角結膜炎	777	□巨細胞	380
□下顎の	289	□関節	722	□巨細胞性エプーリス	510
□下顎隆起	518	□関節炎	591	□巨歯症	986
□核，神経核	808	□関節強直	756	□巨唇症	234
□顎(骨)	84	□関節弛緩	848	□巨人症	945
□顎関節	721	□関節周囲の	732	□巨舌症	248
□角化した	404	□関節痛	585	□巨大歯	37
□角化重層扁平上皮	405	□関節軟骨	725	□筋	229
□角化症	968	□関節軟骨石灰化症	748	□筋緊張	972
□顎下腺	384	□関節の	724	□筋上皮島	478
□角化嚢胞	329	□関節リウマチ	740	□近心頬側の	26
□角化嚢胞性歯原性腫瘍	421	□汗腺	401	□近心舌側の	21
□顎関節症	720	□感染，感染症	292		
□角結膜炎	776	□陥入する	34	**く**	
□角質増殖	633	□顔貌	934		
□核上(性)の	810	□顔面筋，表情筋	807	□クインケ浮腫	602
□拡張	603	□顔面痙攣	820	□くさび状欠損	134
□化合物	51	□顔面神経	688	□口周囲の	544
□過誤腫	995	□顔面神経麻痺	805	□屈曲	980
□過誤腫性の	438	□顔面非対称	719	□クモ指	895
□過剰歯	1	□顔面裂	221	□クラインフェルター症候群	973
□化生	788	□間葉性の	434	□クルーゾン症候群	856
□滑液	751	□乾酪壊死	320		
□合併症	416	□乾酪性の	319	**け**	
□滑膜	729				
□滑膜軟骨腫症	753	**き**		□形成不全，減形成	52
□滑膜の	728			□形成不全の	888
□化膿性関節炎	731	□奇形	29	□痙攣	821
□化膿性の	195,710,734	□義歯	514	□結核	312
□過敏症	142	□義歯性線維腫	513	□結核(性)の	315
□カフェオレ斑	921	□基質	56,452	□結核性頸部リンパ節炎	314
□下部の，下方の	359	□基底細胞	901	□血管	158

143

□血管腫	237,929	□口腔ジスキネジア	826	□腰の，腰椎の	868
□血管性浮腫	601	□口腔粘膜	193	□コステン症候群	736
□血管の	149	□口腔扁平苔癬	621	□骨壊死	715
□結合組織	297	□咬合	95	□骨炎	703
□欠失	982	□硬口蓋	228	□骨化	836
□結晶	747	□高口蓋	275	□骨格	104
□血清，漿液	961	□咬合高径	98	□骨格系	277
□結石	785	□咬合性外傷	204	□骨格の	276
□結節	19	□咬合の	77	□骨吸収	842
□結節性紅斑	614	□咬合平面	78	□骨棘	727
□欠損	853	□咬合面	123	□骨形成性エプーリス	509
□結腸	913	□咬合力	131	□骨形成不全症	844
□欠乏	653	□交叉咬合	85	□骨腫	914
□ケルビズム	529	□好酸性の	471	□骨髄	709
□原因，病因	474	□口臭	182	□骨髄炎	708
□幻影細胞	442	□溝状舌	667	□骨性異形成症	519
□限局性の	113	□甲状舌管	408	□骨内(性)の	427
□犬歯	348	□甲状舌管嚢胞	406	□骨軟骨腫	752
□原始性嚢胞	321	□甲状線，甲状腺の	255	□骨の	922
□倦怠感	583	□甲状腺癌	916	□骨膜	705
□原発性骨内扁平上皮癌	454	□甲状腺機能低下症	236	□骨膜炎	704
□原発性低身長症	931	□甲状腺の	255	□骨密度	841
□原発性の	455	□口唇炎	679	□コプリック斑	560
		□口唇粘膜	680	□コラーゲン	845
		□口唇ヘルペス	542	□孤立性の	375
こ		□口唇裂	208	□根管	954
		□抗精神病薬	828	□根尖	165
□鯉口	935	□硬組織	436	□根尖(部)の	157
□硬化	484	□酵素の	119	□根尖周囲の	365
□口蓋	217	□抗体	996	□根尖性歯周炎	162
□口蓋咽頭の	232	□紅潮	779	□根治手術	417
□口蓋中央の	700	□硬直	733		
□口蓋突起	220	□口底	293		
□口蓋隆起	516	□後天的な，後天性の	240	**さ**	
□口蓋裂	216	□咬頭	22		
□口角	618	□後頭部	979	□再活性化	546
□口角炎	651	□高尿酸血症	745	□鰓弓	872
□口角びらん	650	□紅斑	174	□細菌	711
□高カルシウム血症	964	□紅斑(性)の	666	□細菌(性)の	654
□交感神経の	999	□紅板症	634	□臍帯ヘルニア	944
□口峡	555	□後方の	110	□鰓嚢胞	409
□咬筋	244	□咬耗症	122	□再発(性)の	608
□咬筋肥大症	243	□肛門	579	□再発性アフタ性口内炎	607
□口腔	219	□高リン酸塩尿症	963	□細胞間接着分子	566
□口腔癌	486	□ゴールデンハー症候群	875	□細胞質	469
□口腔カンジダ症	628	□コクサッキーウイルス	554	□鰓裂	412
□口腔乾燥症	760	□黒毛舌	669	□鎖角化の	422
□口腔顔面指趾症候群	881			□鎖骨	835

項目	ページ
☐鎖骨頭蓋異形成症	832
☐鎖骨頭蓋異骨症	833
☐擦過傷	696
☐酸	118
☐三叉神経	793
☐三叉神経痛	790
☐酸蝕症	128
☐残留囊胞	367

し

項目	ページ
☐肢	864
☐歯(性)の	295
☐シェーグレン症候群	775
☐耳介	855
☐耳介前方の	878
☐耳介側頭神経	782
☐歯牙形成	65
☐歯牙腫	437
☐耳下腺	413
☐歯冠	16
☐歯冠周囲炎，智歯周囲炎	281
☐歯間乳頭	184
☐歯冠(部)の	32
☐色素失調症	957
☐色素性母斑	641
☐色素沈着	525
☐色素沈着過剰	648
☐色素沈着過剰の	959
☐色素の沈着した	643
☐シクロスポリン（免疫抑制薬）	273
☐歯頸縁	41
☐歯頸部	207
☐歯頸(部)の，頸部の	40
☐刺激性物質	690
☐歯原性角化囊胞	328
☐歯原性線維腫	443
☐歯原性粘液腫	448
☐歯原性囊胞	323
☐歯垢，プラーク	168
☐自己抗体	565
☐自己免疫疾患	564
☐自己免疫の	563
☐歯根	17
☐歯根吸収	159
☐歯根の	363

項目	ページ
☐歯根囊胞	362
☐歯根膜	342
☐歯周炎	163
☐歯周靭帯	202
☐歯周組織	197
☐歯周の	164
☐歯周囊胞	368
☐歯周ポケット	199
☐思春期	528
☐思春期早発症	527
☐糸状乳頭	664
☐歯小囊	446
☐歯髄	148
☐歯髄壊死	152
☐歯髄炎	151
☐歯髄腔	35
☐歯髄結石	144
☐歯髄充血	146
☐ジスキネジア	827
☐歯性上顎洞炎	301
☐歯性扁桃周囲炎	294
☐歯石	198,988
☐脂腺	400
☐歯槽	140
☐歯槽骨	201
☐歯槽骨炎	702
☐歯槽突起	215
☐歯槽粘膜	340
☐歯槽の	200
☐歯槽裂，顎裂	214
☐失活歯	366
☐実質	479
☐膝神経節	814
☐歯堤	262
☐歯内歯	28
☐歯肉	167
☐歯肉縁	137
☐歯肉炎	166
☐歯肉口内炎	535
☐歯肉線維腫症	263
☐歯肉増殖	268
☐歯肉退縮	206
☐歯肉の	136
☐歯肉膿瘍	187
☐歯乳囊胞	345
☐歯乳頭	445
☐歯胚	12

項目	ページ
☐脂肪類皮腫	877
☐斜顔(面)裂	225
☐灼熱痛	739
☐斜指	892
☐斜視	984
☐充血	147
☐集合性歯牙腫	439
☐収縮	823
☐重層扁平上皮	332
☐18トリソミー症候群	977
☐手術，外科的処置	418
☐手掌	904
☐腫脹	170
☐出血	171,371
☐術後性上顎囊胞	415
☐腫瘍	250
☐上咽頭収縮筋	233
☐漿液(性)の	502
☐小窩	903
☐上下顎前突	106
☐上顎(骨)	91
☐上顎(骨)の	5
☐小顎症	879
☐上顎前突症	103
☐上顎洞	303
☐上顎突起	212
☐小臼歯	349
☐小結節	46
☐小結節性の	313
☐症候群	523
☐小口症	241
☐小歯症	985
☐症状	582
☐小水疱	543
☐小水疱(性)の	536
☐小舌症	252
☐常染色体(性)の	882
☐小帯	280
☐小頭症	971
☐上皮	334
☐上皮(性)の	258
☐上皮真珠	257
☐上部の，上方の	218
☐静脈の	372
☐小葉	789
☐食欲不振	649
☐女性化乳房	976

語	番号
歯蕾	435
歯列弓	72
歯瘻	191
神経	552
神経障害性の	802
神経節	815
神経線維腫	920
神経線維腫症1型	919
神経痛	791
神経痛の	549
神経堤	873
心血管の	896
滲出	735
滲出物	610
浸潤	477
浸潤性の	450
尋常性狼瘡	309
新生児	260
新生児の	80
新生物	488
腎臓の	594
唇側の	86
靭帯	203
真皮	685
心膜炎	593

す

語	番号
水癌	616
髄室	953
水晶体偏位	899
水痘・帯状疱疹ウイルス	548
水疱	568
水疱(性)の	588
スタージ・ウェーバー症候群	923
頭痛	584
スティーヴンズ・ジョンソン症候群	577

せ

語	番号
正角化の	331
生活歯	344
静止性骨空洞	381
脆弱性	846
生殖器	580

語	番号
生殖器の，陰部の	612
精神遅滞	927
精巣	974
正中顔面裂	223
正中頸嚢胞	407
正中歯	2
正中の	222
正中菱形舌炎	674
赤唇縁	681
脊柱の	880
舌咽神経	797
舌咽神経痛	796
切縁	42
舌炎	661
石灰化	327
石灰化した	145
石灰化上皮性歯原性腫瘍	426
石灰化嚢胞性歯原性腫瘍	441
舌下腺	393
舌下の	290
舌甲状腺	254
舌根	799
舌根沈下	948
切痕のある	67
切歯	7
切歯管	357
舌小帯	279
舌小帯短縮症	278
接触性口唇炎	689
舌側の	20
切端咬合	96
舌痛症	803
舌扁桃	678
舌扁桃肥大	677
舌裂	253
セメントエナメル境	47
セメント芽細胞腫	453
セメント質	14
腺	385
腺(性)の	351
線維芽細胞(性)の	444
線維骨性の	521
線維腫	433
線維腫症	264
線維腫性エプーリス	508
線維性結合組織	447
線維性の	266

語	番号
線維肉腫	460
前癌性の	632
前歯	90
腺腫	463
腺腫様歯原性腫瘍	423
栓状歯	39
染色体	938
全身症状	712
全身性エリテマトーデス	590
全身(性)の	581,840
腺性歯原性嚢胞	350
前舌腺	396
腺組織	496
先天歯	79
先天性エプーリス	512
先天性外胚葉形成不全，先天性外胚葉異形成症	956
先天性鼻咽腔閉鎖不全症	231
先天的な，先天性の	9
尖頭合指症	862
尖頭歯	992
前頭隆起	866
尖部	395
潜伏(性)の	547
腺房細胞	503
腺房細胞癌	500
腺房の	485
前方の	89
腺様嚢胞癌	490
前彎	869

そ

語	番号
早期萌出	987
象牙質	11
象牙質異形成症	951
象牙質形成不全症	950
象牙質知覚過敏症	141
象牙質粒	143
増殖	428
増殖，過形成	267
増殖(物)	506
叢生	101
双生歯	15
僧房弁逸脱	898
掻痒性の	572
側頭嚢胞	410

□側切歯	31
□足底	905
□側方性歯周嚢胞	341
□組織	75
□組織学の	491
□咀嚼	794
□損傷，外傷	205

た

□ターナー歯	60
□ターナー症候群	936
□第一大臼歯	70
□第一第二鰓弓症候群	871
□大臼歯	23
□対合歯	92
□第三大臼歯	282
□代謝	744
□代謝性の	271
□帯状疱疹	545
□苔癬	622
□大泉門	933
□大動脈解離	897
□大脳	811
□大脳鎌	906
□大理石骨病	838,839
□タウロドント	43
□ダウン症候群	969
□唾液	763
□唾液管炎	768
□唾液腺	464
□唾液腺炎	482,765
□唾液腺化生	787
□唾液瘻	759
□多核(性)の	379
□多形紅斑	574
□多形腺腫	462
□多系統(性)の	894
□多骨性線維性異形成症	524
□唾石	766
□唾石症	783
□脱臼	139
□(壊死部分が)脱落する	183
□多発性の	259
□多病巣性の	532
□多房性の	353
□短指	891

□単純性骨嚢胞	369
□単純ヘルペスウイルス	540
□炭水化物	121
□単病巣性の	531
□単房性の	352
□短腕	983

ち

□智歯	299
□地図状舌	672
□中間細胞	499
□中心咬合位	94
□中切歯	6
□中毒性表皮壊死症	586
□腸管	910
□長骨	377
□貯留嚢胞	389
□沈着	639
□沈着物	430

つ

□椎骨	378
□痛風	742
□つま楊枝	126

て

□手足口病	558
□低悪性度の	501
□低位咬合	97
□低位歯	76
□低血圧	647
□低血糖	946
□低出生体重	932
□低身長	939
□低身長症	865
□低フォスファターゼ症	960
□デスモイド腫瘍	917
□鉄欠乏性貧血	659
□転位	71
□てんかん	926
□伝染性の	772
□デンタルフロス	127
□天疱瘡	562

と

□頭蓋	837,915
□頭蓋顔面異骨症	857
□頭蓋底	108
□頭蓋の	107
□頭蓋縫合早期癒合症	858
□透過性	604
□導管	390
□導管周囲の	483
□疼痛	173
□頭皮	597
□動脈瘤	993
□動脈瘤の	374
□動揺	955
□特発性の	673
□ドライマウス	761
□トリーチャー・コリンズ症候群	849

な

□内側の	210
□内反膝	870
□内部吸収	161
□内分泌の	251
□軟口蓋	230
□軟骨	726
□軟骨(性)の	755
□軟骨腫(症)	754
□軟骨石灰化(症)	749
□軟骨無形成症	863
□軟組織	190
□難聴	737
□軟膜の	928

に

□肉芽腫	318
□肉芽腫性エプーリス	507
□肉芽腫性口唇炎	682
□ニコチン性口内炎	637
□21トリソミー症候群	970
□二重唇	239
□ニフェジピン（血圧降下薬）	274
□二分肋骨	907

□乳歯	63	□歯が生える	694	□表皮水疱症	573
□乳児	695	□歯ぎしり	132	□表皮の	587
□乳腺	493	□白板症	631	□病変	135
□乳頭	185	□剥離	177,589	□鼻翼	360
□乳頭(状)の	466	□剥離性歯肉炎	172	□鼻翼軟骨	889
□尿酸ナトリウム	746	□破骨細胞	843	□びらん	537
□二裂舌	886	□破折	138	□びらん(性)の	627
□妊娠性エプーリス	511	□発育障害	55	□鼻梁	890
		□発汗	780	□鼻涙管	361
ね		□抜歯	300	□ピロリン酸カルシウム	750
		□ハッチンソン歯	66	□貧血	595
□猫鳴き症候群	981	□発痛点	795		
□練り歯磨き	133	□発熱	58	**ふ**	
□粘液	492	□パピヨン・ルフェーヴル症候群	967		
□粘液細胞	497			□フェニトイン(抗痙攣薬)	272
□粘液腫	449	□歯ブラシ	125	□フォーダイス斑	676
□粘液腺	391	□パラミクソウイルス	773	□フォン・レックリングハウゼン病	918
□粘液の	388	□斑	598,626		
□粘液嚢胞	386	□瘢痕	600	□副交感神経の	781
□粘液様の	451	□斑状歯	53	□複合性局所疼痛症候群	801
□粘液瘤	387	□ハンター舌炎	663	□複雑性歯牙腫	440
□捻転	102			□副作用	716
□粘表皮癌	495	**ひ**		□副腎皮質の	645
□粘膜	194,569			□副唾液腺	757
□粘膜下口蓋裂	226	□ピエール・ロバン症候群	947	□副鼻腔炎	302
□粘膜下の	227	□非炎症性の	265	□浮腫	249
□粘膜と皮膚の	571	□皮下組織	286	□浮腫(性)の	575
□粘膜の	175	□皮下の	285	□不随意の	822
		□非乾酪性の	683	□不正咬合	83
の		□鼻孔	578	□不全麻痺	806
		□鼻口蓋管	356	□付属器	399
□膿	189	□鼻口蓋管嚢胞	355	□付着歯肉	347
□脳幹	812	□鼻歯槽嚢胞	358	□フッ素	50
□脳神経	824	□ビスフォスフォネート	714	□フッ素症	49
□嚢胞	322	□ビスフォスフォネート関連顎骨壊死	713	□ぶどう酒様血管腫	924
□嚢胞の, 嚢胞性の	324			□ブドウ膜炎	613
□膿瘍	188	□微生物	120	□不妊	941
		□肥大	245	□フライ症候群	778
は		□ビタミン	665	□ブランダン・ヌーン嚢胞	394
		□鼻突起	211	□プランマー・ヴィンソン症候群	658
□背(部)	671	□皮膚	284		
□背(部)の	668	□皮膚炎	657	□プリン	743
□敗血症	308	□皮膚の	311	□フルニエ歯	68
□梅毒	59	□びまん性の	269	□フレンジ, 義歯床翼部	515
□胚の	213	□病的骨折	965	□プロトスタイリッド	24
□排膿瘻孔	307	□病的な, 病理学(上)の	784	□分化	504
□胚発生	414	□表皮	997	□分岐部	48

項目	ページ
□分子	567
□分泌	762
□分泌不全	767
□分葉舌	885

へ

項目	ページ
□平滑舌	662
□閉塞	156,952
□ベーチェット病	611
□ベックウィズ・ヴィーデマン症候群	942
□ベドナー・アフタ	697
□ヘルパンギーナ	553
□ヘルペス	539
□ヘルペス(性)の	534
□ヘルペス性歯肉口内炎,疱疹性歯肉口内炎	533
□ベル麻痺	818
□偏位	87
□辺縁歯肉	186
□辺縁性歯周炎	304
□変形	741
□変形性関節症	723
□片側の	246
□変色	670
□変性	325
□扁桃	298
□扁桃炎	991
□扁桃周囲炎	296
□扁平上皮	333
□扁平上皮細胞	456
□扁平苔癬	623

ほ

項目	ページ
□ポイツ・ジェガース症候群	908
□蜂窩織炎, 蜂巣炎	283
□萌出	82
□萌出した	3
□萌出する	74
□萌出遅延	81
□萌出嚢胞	339
□膨疹	606
□縫線	701
□放線菌症	305
□放線菌属	306

項目	ページ
□発作(性)の	792
□発疹	550
□発赤	169
□母斑	642
□ポリープ	912
□ポリープ症	909

ま

項目	ページ
□埋伏歯	73
□膜	343
□麻疹	561
□マッキューン・オールブライト症候群	687,819
□末梢(性)の	809
□麻痺	
□摩耗症	124
□マルファン症候群	893
□慢性硬化性顎下腺炎	480
□慢性歯周炎	196
□慢性歯髄炎	155
□慢性の	154

み

項目	ページ
□味覚	830
□味覚異常	829
□味覚消失	804
□ミクリッツ病	774
□ミトコンドリア	472
□未萌出の	4
□耳鳴り	738
□脈瘤性骨嚢胞	373

む

項目	ページ
□ムーン歯	69
□無機の	115
□無歯症	8
□無症候性の	382
□無精子症	975

め

項目	ページ
□迷入唾液腺	758
□めまい	816
□メラニン	640

項目	ページ
□メラニン沈着	638
□メルカーソン・ローゼンタール症候群	686

も

項目	ページ
□毛細血管	605
□網状の	624
□毛状白板症	635
□毛包	402

や

項目	ページ
□薬物性口内炎	619

ゆ

項目	ページ
□有郭乳頭	675
□有機酸	117
□有機の	116
□優性の	902
□遊走する	874
□遊離歯肉	346
□癒合歯	10
□癒着歯	13

よ

項目	ページ
□溶解	114
□溶骨性の	376
□翼状頸	940

ら

項目	ページ
□ラッセル・シルヴァー症候群	930
□ラムゼイ・ハント症候群	813
□ランゲルハンス細胞組織球症	530

り

項目	ページ
□リガ・フェーデ病	692
□裏装する	330
□隆起	517
□流行性耳下腺炎	769
□流行性の, 流行	771

- 流涎症 764
- 両眼隔離 859
- 良性の 370
- 良性リンパ上皮性病変 473
- 両側の 247
- 緑内障 925
- リンパ管腫 238
- リンパ球 476
- リンパ上皮性囊胞 411
- リンパ節 317
- リンパ節炎 316
- リンパ組織 467

る

- 類上皮細胞 684
- 涙腺 475
- 類天疱瘡 570
- 類皮囊胞 397
- 類表皮細胞 498
- 類表皮囊胞 403
- ルートヴィヒアンギナ 287

れ

- 裂 209
- 劣性の 883

ろ

- 瘻孔 192
- 狼瘡 310
- 濾胞性歯囊胞 336
- 濾胞性の,小胞性の 337

わ

- 矮小歯 36

■著者略歴■

近藤真治（こんどう　しんじ）

1965年米国カリフォルニア州生まれ．上智大学外国語学部英語学科卒業．ミシガン州立大学大学院コミュニケーション研究科修士課程修了．岐阜経済大学経済学部専任講師，福井大学医学部助教授，同教授を経て，現在は愛知医科大学看護学部教授（医療英語）．主な著書に，『コミュニケーション不安の形成と治療』（共著，ナカニシヤ出版），『からだの英語集中マスター』（共著，メジカルビュー社），『その症候，英語で言えますか？』（羊土社），『生物学英単語500』（三修社）など．

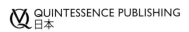

疾患別 歯学英単語1000

2017年11月10日　第1版第1刷発行

著　　者　近藤真治

発 行 人　北峯康充

発 行 所　クインテッセンス出版株式会社
東京都文京区本郷3丁目2番6号　〒113-0033
クイントハウスビル　電話(03)5842-2270(代表)
(03)5842-2272(営業部)
(03)5842-2275(編集部)
web page address　http://www.quint-j.co.jp/

印刷・製本　サン美術印刷株式会社

©2017　クインテッセンス出版株式会社　　　　　　　　禁無断転載・複写
Printed in Japan　　　　　　　　　　　　　　　落丁本・乱丁本はお取り替えします
ISBN978-4-7812-0584-7　C3047　　　　　　　定価はカバーに表示してあります